The A–Z of Community Mental Health Practice

Edited by

Sheila Forster

Stanley Thornes (Publishers) Ltd

First published in 1997 by:
Stanley Thornes (Publishers) Ltd
Ellenborough House
Wellington Street
CHELTENHAM
GL50 1YW
United Kingdom

97 98 99 00 01 / 10 9 8 7 6 5 4 3 2 1

A catalogue record for this book is available from the British
Library

Library of Congress Catalog Card Number: 96-72124

ISBN 0-7487-3175-X

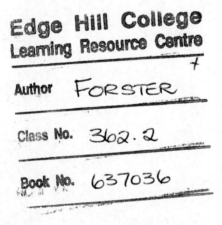
Distributed in the USA and Canada by Singular Publishing Group
Inc., 4284 41st Street, San Diego, California 92105

Typeset by Mews Photosetting, Beckenham, Kent
Printed in Great Britain by T. J. International Ltd

Contents

Contributors	ix
Preface	xi
Acknowledgements	xii
Access to Health Records Act 1990	1
Access to services in the community	1
Accountability	2
Action plans	5
Addiction services	6
Admission	6
Advocacy	7
Aims of visits	8
Alerts and emergencies	10
Anxiety management	11
Appointments	12
Assessment	13
Behavioural psychotherapy	17
Bereavement	18
Boundary setting	20
Care Programme Approach (CPA)	23
Carers	25
Case management	26
Clinical audit	27
Clinical supervision	28

Closures   29
Communication and relationship-building techniques – different
      approaches to the therapeutic relationship   30
Confidentiality   31
Coping and violence   31
Crisis intervention   32
Crisis intervention teams and crisis response teams   33

Data Protection Act 1984   35
Day care facilities   36
Delusions   37
Depression   39
Diffusing anger   41
Discharge from hospital   42
Disorientation   43
Documentation   44
Drama techniques   48

Elderly mental health services   49
Emotional effects of physical illness   50
Empowerment   51
Evaluation   51

Family therapy   53

Getting in (initial visit)   55
Goal setting   56

Hallucinations   59
Health of the nation   61
HIV positive and hepatitis B – administration of medicine   61
HIV/AIDS and mental health   62
Housing   63

Implementation   65
Individual performance review   66
Information technology   66
Institutional behaviour   68
Intervention styles   69
Interviews   70

Knowing your patch   73

Labelling   75
Learned helplessness   76
Legal vulnerability   76
Life events   77

Management supervision   79
Managing manipulation   80
Mania   81
Medication and mental health   83
Mental Health Act 1983   84
Mental Health Act Code of Practice   85
Mental Health Bill 1995   87
Mental health promotion   88
Mother and baby – postnatal mental health needs   90
Multidisciplinary teams   91

Normalization – social role valorization   93
Non-verbal communication   95

Observation and monitoring   97
Obstacles   97
Outcomes of care   98

Patient or client?   101
Patient's Charter   102
Problem solving process   103
Professional development   103
Projection   104
Psychosomatic illness   105

Quality assurance   107

Rational emotive therapy   109
Referral process   109
Reflective practice   110
Relationship-building skills   111
Relaxation techniques   112
Reminiscence therapy and reality orientation   113
Resource centres   114

Schizophrenia   117
Self-help groups   119
Setting up supervision   120
Sexuality   121
Sexual problems   122
Side effects of medication   123
Social skills training   124
Standard of care   124
Stress and coping   125
Stressors and community mental health care   127
Students   129
Supervision register   130

viii **Contents**

Terminating a relationship   133
Transcultural issues in mental health care   133
Transference and counter-transference   135

Women and mental health   137
Working base   138
Working in partnership – collaborative approach to care   139

Appendix   143
References   147
Further reading   153

Contributors

Sheila Forster Cert Ed, BEd, RMN, CPN Cert, RNT, MEd, Dip Couns
Sheila Forster initially trained as a secondary school teacher but retrained a few years later and qualified as a psychiatric nurse in 1983 at St Augustine's Hospital, Canterbury. She then worked as a Community Psychiatric Nurse in Kent for five years before moving to nurse education in 1989. She now works at Canterbury Christ Church College as a Senior Lecturer specializing in the teaching of interpersonal skills, retaining her interest in and contact with the field of community mental health work.

Alan Cullen RMN, CPN Cert
Alan Cullen began his mental health nurse training in 1975 at St Augustine's Hospital, Canterbury and commenced generic CPN working in 1980. In 1987 he took up the joint post of CPN/Nurse Teacher. He remained in this post for three years before deciding to return to his main interest, the mental health needs of the elderly. He is currently a Community Psychiatric Nurse employed by the South Kent Community Healthcare NHS Trust. His catchment area, Dover, Deal and Folkestone, has an elderly population higher than the national average and it is in this client group that he has specialized for the past six years.

Charles Flynn BSc, RMN, RGN
Charles Flynn trained as a registered mental nurse and registered general nurse at the Renfrew, Dumbarton and Argyll College of Nursing and Midwifery, Paisley, Scotland in the early 1980s. He then worked in London for a period, mainly in acute psychiatry and the mental health care of

elderly people, before moving into senior management posts. He is currently Director of Clinical Services and Executive Nurse with Southport and Formby Community Health Services NHS Trust. His interests lie in the development of holistic models of care which genuinely involve service users and carers.

Hilary McCallion RMN, BA(Hons), Diploma in Nursing Studies, Certificate in Counselling Skills
Hilary McCallion worked in community mental health for a number of years before moving into education. She has been employed by Pathfinder Mental Health Services NHS Trust since November 1994 as Assistant Director of Nursing, Professional Development. Her main interests include the politics of mental health care, the future of nursing and caring as healing. She has recently been awarded a Florence Nightingale Award to study AIDS-related brain impairment in the USA and the UK.

Contributions have also been gratefully received from:
Thomas McCallion, Community Psychiatric Nurse, South London; Colin McCarthy, Principal Lecturer, Mental Health, Chester College; Nicola Ramsey, Assistant Director of Nursing, Pathfinder Trust; John Soanes, Project Worker, Pathfinder Trust; Catherine Wells, Clinical Nurse Specialist in Behavioural Psychotherapy, City and Hackney Community Services Trust; Chris Willets, Course Co-ordinator (learning disability), Canterbury Christ Church College.

Preface

The impetus behind this book came not only from personal experiences as mental health nurses working in the community but also through feedback from students spending time in the community, who commonly returned to college with comments about practical difficulties that they had not foreseen, and their awareness that they had underestimated the value that is ascribed to the visitor by the client. We have attempted in this text to address two main issues. First, when working in the community, what are the practical issues that arise and how can they be overcome? These may range from the experience of aggression occurring in someone's home to taking a life history assessment. Second, how can the therapeutic presence of the practitioner be maximized to the advantage of the client, and what are the theories and skills available to ensure this?

Although this book is written from a nursing perspective, it is intended that much of the material included will be equally applicable to any community practitioner, particularly those working in multidisciplinary teams who share many of the same issues and difficulties.

We wrote this book intending it to be used by professionals with varying levels of experience, who needed information quickly about a wide variety of subjects that are applicable to working in the community. It is therefore a 'dip into' book which hopefully will come to be an essential item in each professional's back pocket or brief case!

Sheila Forster (editor)
Canterbury, August 1996

Acknowledgements

The idea for the creation of this book came from a long conversation with Rosemary Morris, of Chapman & Hall. Her support and humour since then has been invaluable, plus her faith in the success of this book at times when I had lost sight of it.

My first exposure to the theory behind community work came from Tony Leiba, whose vision of community mental health practice excited me when I was a CPN, and whose enthusiasm has always since then been contagious.

Thanks are especially due to the contributors to this book for the amount of hard work and energy that they showed. Alan Cullen, supported by Carol, was in this venture from the beginning, and the knowledge and expertise that he has gained from many years of practising in the community has been invaluable. Working so closely with the principal contributors has been an uplifting experience.

Many people have showed interest and given support in various ways, including Bill and Helen Forster, and Karl Williams, which has often kept me going.

And finally, enormous thanks to Chris, who not only lent me full secretarial and computer facilities, but also has put up uncomplainingly with the disruption to our lives caused by the writing of this book, and will enjoy celebrating the return to normality!

A

ACCESS TO HEALTH RECORDS ACT 1990 (*see also* Confidentiality; Data Protection Act 1984)

This Act covers the disclosure of manually-held personal health information, as opposed to information that is held on a computer. A wide variety of health care professionals can disclose the information required, excluding social workers. The same exclusions apply as for the Data Protection Act. Inaccuracies in the information disclosed must be corrected and anything that is unintelligible, such as technical terms or jargon, must be explained to the client.

ACCESS TO SERVICES IN THE COMMUNITY (*see also* Resource Centres)

Services for clients who have experienced mental health problems in the community are as well developed today as they ever have been. At the same time, however, those same services are under pressure as never before. Expectations of all service providers have been raised by a series of charters, which seem to indicate to some service consumers that they have the right to demand services. At the same time, legislation such as the NHS and Community Care Act 1990 and subsequent caselaw clearly indicates that there is a financial limit to resources which are being provided by the Government for community-based services.

Services in the community have never been evenly distributed. A day service which is provided by the social services department in one area may not be known in another. Access to services is also limited. Some service providers take care to publicize the services which they are providing.

Others may take a much lower profile, and attempt to minimize new demand. Charges for services may also have the same impact, especially when they are imposed on a previously free service. The Black Report (1980) is well known to have shown up social class divisions in health service access in the UK, with evidence being provided that the higher the social class of an individual, the better was access to health services.

Clients with mental health problems and their carers face particular difficulties in accessing services. Often individual motivation and ability to investigate and access services may be impaired as part of the illness. In addition, considerable evidence exists (Verbrugge, 1985) for a gender bias to poor health, which is matched by the higher ratio of women to men experiencing mental health problems over their lifetime.

A number of issues arise for the practitioner working in the community as a consequence of these issues. It is important that the practitioner is aware of what is available in their local area, taking into account particular patterns of service provision. Services need to be accessible to individuals from all communities, including ethnic minority groups, and particular care may need to be taken to ensure that this is possible. While it is clearly impossible for every practitioner to know about every service, it is important that the individual working in the community is able to get accurate up-to-date information as soon as possible. Where a particular service is needed and is not available, the individual practitioner should make the need known to the relevant authority. Indeed, it may sometimes be possible for the practitioner to assist in the establishment of such a service, either facilitating such action, or working directly to ensure it is provided. It needs to be recognized that, at times, there is a danger to the practitioner following this approach. Most practitioners are employees, and may be required to follow particular policies relating to their employment. Clearly the clients' interests require that their needs are properly and openly put to the relevant agencies. This is probably best done by assisting clients or their carers to access an independent advocacy service.

The appropriate and proper provision of care in the community requires that clients who need services can access them. Practitioners working in the community need to be sensitive to the ongoing and changing needs of individuals and groups in the community.

ACCOUNTABILITY

Community care involves providing a range of services which suits the individual's needs. It has been argued that care should be user-led based on their wishes and culture and not be determined by the service (Payne, 1986).

To provide a range of services and seamless care, multidisciplinary teams have emerged to ensure that the necessary range of skills is available to ensure a comprehensive package of care. What all disciplines have in common is the object of serving the interests of those in their care, that is to cause no harm, to ensure standards are maintained and to respect patients' rights. At times these values may be tested in view of organisational changes, manpower availability, accessibility to services, financial restrictions and the law.

Although the focus of care in today's health service advocates client choice and collaboration, at times conflict can arise due to requirements of Acts of Parliament, for instance The Mental Health Act 1983 or common law, that is the duty of care. Professionals may have to make decisions which on the surface may be contrary to the expressed wishes of clients, but because of their responsibilities to higher authorities, the law or ethical and moral responsibilities, their control and ability to take charge of client care is removed. However, professionals will always be expected to account for their practice and justify why and how decisions were made, given the circumstances and parameters within which they work. They are also expected to account for their actions in terms of the standards of care set by their governing body, employers, society, the client and themselves.

The following text describes in detail accountability as applied to the nurse, but is equally relevant to all professionals responsible for delivering care.

Nurses are professional practitioners and as such are individually accountable for their actions and omissions. Accountability means not only having to answer for an action when something goes wrong, but also involves a continuous process of monitoring how they perform professionally. A nurse's responsibility differs in different situations but they need to be aware that they are constantly responsible and therefore constantly accountable (Tschudin, 1986). Accountability cannot be delegated to another or avoided: responsibilities can be delegated but the registered nurse remains accountable.

To have responsibility means to respond or to answer to someone or something (Tschudin, 1986). Thompson *et al.* (1988) distinguish between four types of responsibilities:

1. responsibility for one's own action (personal responsibility);
2. responsibility for the care of someone (fiduciary responsibility);
3. responsibility to a higher authority (professional accountability);
4. responsibility to the wider society (public accountability).

The UKCC *Code of Professional Conduct* (1984) and *Exercising Accountability* (1989) indicates nurses are primarily accountable to the client and public. However, it has been argued that nurses are also accountable to the employer, profession and self (Tingle, 1990).

Professional accountability

A registered nurse is an autonomous practitioner; to be autonomous one has to have the freedom and authority to act. In practice this means as a professional 'you have the ability to make direct and independent decisions in the nursing care of patients, which the nurse may consider to be solely within her domain' (Copp, 1986). You will also be expected to explain and/or be answerable for those decisions (Carpenter, 1993; Carlisle, 1990; UKCC, 1989).

Personal accountability

Nurses have to live with the decisions they make and not allow personal views to affect adversely the care they deliver.

Organizational accountability

Nurses are employed on the basis of a job description which outlines the practitioner's roles and responsibilities. The nurse is accountable to the employer for carrying out the tasks and duties specified by the organization (Hyde, 1985; Rhodes, 1983). Job descriptions are generally designed to take account of the profession's code of conduct and it is highly unlikely an employer would expect a nurse to practise in such a way as to jeopardize the interests of the client.

Accountability is to the client and should circumstances arise where a potential or actual breach of the code of conduct occurs, the nurse is responsible for informing those who are empowered to resolve the situation (Carpenter, 1993).

Client and public accountability

The code of professional conduct states the duties of the registered nurse in which care can be measured. There are expectations and standards which a registered nurse is expected to achieve and comply with. Breach of these will result in professional misconduct.

Finally, there is a relationship between accountability and the law. The nurse is liable for any acts or omissions which cause harm to the client. The client can sue for negligence, which is damage caused by the breach of a duty to care (Tingle, 1990). Dimond (1990, page 5) outlines four arenas of accountability in which the nurse can be held in law to explain their actions:

1. public – criminal law;
2. client – civil law;

3. profession – governing body (UKCC);
4. employer – contract of employment (industrial tribunal).

ACTION PLANS

Producing action plans can be a useful strategy for community mental health nurses when they find themselves faced with complex issues. The technique is equally useful for clinical, administrative or managerial issues. The purpose of an action plan is to sub-divide a problem into discrete sub-objectives which can then be arranged in a logical sequence. This will give a chronological hierarchy of the sub-objectives which, on completion of the last sub-objective, should satisfy the overall task.

Action plans should not contain detailed rationale for the proposed actions. Such explanations would only distract attention from the key issues, that is what needs to be done, by whom and by when. Where an action plan requires the contribution of a number of individuals or organizations it is essential that these individuals or organizations are aware of what is required of them and agree to complete the actions in the agreed timescale.

Action plans are working documents allowing progress to be monitored towards the final objective. Completion dates for each sub-objective should be used as review dates for the entire action plan, allowing confirmation or revision of the timescale and sub-objectives in the light of experience to that date. This discipline ensures that the action plan remains a live document rather than becoming the sole objective in itself. Such tokenism can be avoided by describing the formulation of the action plan as the first objective of the action plan.

Action plans usually have three columns but occasionally four: these are headed action, lead responsibility and completion date. A typical example would be an action plan arising from a complex case review where a range of objectives have been set for the various agencies contributing to the client's care. Each objective would be written across the full width of the page which would then be sub-divided into three columns and headed appropriately. The sequence of actions necessary to achieve the overall objective could then be formulated and listed chronologically, lead responsibility would be allocated and a realistic timescale set. This should be repeated for each objective. Where there is only one action or a few actions for each objective four columns may be used with the objective being written in the first column. The columns would be headed objective, action, lead responsibility and completion date.

Each action plan is unique, a bespoke tool to achieve specific objectives. It will only be useful if sufficient care is taken when formulating these sub-objectives and where the parties allocated lead responsibility are signed up to delivering and delivering on time.

Action plan formats

Objective		
Action	Lead responsibility	Completion date

Objective	Action	Lead responsibility	Completion date

ADDICTION SERVICES

Within each region will be a specialist service specifically for people with addictions. These services will offer expert advice to generic community mental health workers as well as managing their own caseload of clients with addiction difficulties. Substance abuse and alcohol abuse are usually separated with specialist workers in each. The teams tend to be multi-professional and include nurses, doctors, occupational therapists, social workers and psychologists. Depending on the policy of the team, referrals will be through general practitioners, psychiatrists, professionals in community mental health teams and from the client themselves.

The working practice is specific to each team but in the main the intention is to offer advice, information, education, counselling, home detoxification, group work and referral to dry hostels or hospital units. This may take place at the client's home, health centres, drop-in centres and resource centres. Hospitalization is necessary at times depending on the resources available and the client's needs. Health education is an important part of the work, and needle-exchange schemes are an example of this. Dirty and used needles and syringes can be exchanged for clean material. This is to reduce the risk of infection from AIDS and hepatitis, and often members of the addiction team will have specialist knowledge and offer counselling to the clients on this area. These services are operated in the strictest confidence, but advice and information is on hand should the client require it.

ADMISSION (*see also* The Mental Health Act 1983; Discharge from hospital)

There will be times when a client from the community mental health practitioner's caseload requires admission into a psychiatric hospital. The admission may be planned and brought about by recognition that the client needs more intensive assessment and treatment than can be given in the community setting. Conversely, the admission may be arranged urgently due to a sudden exacerbation of the client's symptoms and/or a deterioration in their social situation. Clients may be admitted voluntarily as informal patients or involuntarily as formal patients under a section of The Mental Health Act 1983. They may be distressed by the admission or relieved, depending on their circumstances and perception of the problem. Practitioners have a role in preparing clients for admission. It can be reassuring for the client to know what to expect, what they will need to take, and when their relatives can visit. Family and carers will also need support and information. Any package of care in place may well include input from formal carers, including care managers and wardens, or informal carers such as good neighbours. Carers will appreciate being informed about the situation and therefore feel more valued and willing to reinstate the care package when the client returns home. This information may be limited to stating that the client is to be admitted into hospital, so will not be requiring care at home for a while. Practitioners should be aware of the need to respect client confidentiality when talking to carers.

The admission will probably have been arranged by the client's general practitioner (GP) and/or consultant psychiatrist. If a section under The Mental Health Act is implemented, then an approved social worker will also be involved. Although the practitioner may not be directly involved with the statutory aspects of the section procedure, the relationship between the client and the practitioner can become strained at these times and a rebuilding of the trusting relationship may need to be undertaken.

It is usual for the client to be allocated a keyworker on the ward, but continuity of care can be enhanced by the community practitioner liaising with this keyworker. By visiting the client on the ward the relationship with the practitioner can continue and trust can be maintained. By attending the ward meetings, the practitioner can provide the team with helpful information and gain feedback on a client's progress. When discharge is being planned, the practitioner is in an ideal position to liaise with carers and assist in the transfer of care from hospital to home. When an admission is necessary, the practitioner may experience a feeling of failure and ask themselves: 'was I skilled enough?' or 'should I have visited more often?' It is worth reminding ourselves that the old negative perception of hospital versus community is fast diminishing and a more positive attitude – the hospital is **in** the community and is a community resource to be used for the benefit of the client – now prevails.

ADVOCACY

Part of the role of a practitioner in community mental health care is to incorporate the role of advocate into the overall work. An advocate can be described as a person who effectively represents the interests of another person who has substantial needs which are unmet and likely to remain unmet without special representation. It is the process of acting for, or on behalf of, someone who is unable to do so for themselves. In mental health care advocacy is essentially about being a representative for people who experience enduring mental illness and who have a right to all the services received by others.

This role could involve upholding rights of the client, acting in the best interests of the client and acting as an intermediary between client and statutory/voluntary services. It is through these endeavours that the community mental health practitioner seeks to improve the client's quality of life. The practitioner is enabling the client to empower themselves to control their own affairs and gain deserved rights.

The role of advocate is non-confrontational and avoids conflict; it is based on an equal relationship and is about enabling people to take a more active role in planning their future.

There are four main issues which underpin the role of the community practitioner working as a client advocate:

1. the quality of care a client receives;
2. their access to care;
3. fully informing clients about the care offered and received;
4. awareness of alternatives to care.

To enable a community mental health practitioner to advocate for another requires knowledge of the client, insight into their needs and their perception of their needs, excellent communication skills, and the ability to listen and hear what the client is saying. Consideration of whether the community mental health practitioner is best placed to be an advocate is necessary especially if this creates conflict with his employing authority. Self-advocacy is vital and this can be achieved by the community mental health practitioner informing and ensuring understanding, teaching assertiveness and problem solving skills, arranging opportunities for clients to discuss issues of their choice.

Advocacy services may be supplied from independent advocates. These independent advocates may be persons who have not had mental health problems but may speak on their behalf. Alternatively, User Advocacy Networks and Patient Councils offer a model of advocacy where the advocates have experienced mental health problems.

AIMS OF VISITS (*see also* Family therapy; Relationship-building skills)

When visiting a client in their own home for the first time, the mental health practitioner will need to have in mind a set of aims. The referrer may have asked for the client to receive support, counselling, a particular therapy or medication and/or have their mental health monitored. However, it is more usual for an assessment to be required initially so that the referrer can be advised on treatment options. Although the practitioner will have in hand the referrer's view of the problem, the view of the client will take priority when designing the care plan. The views of the client's family and carers will be very helpful in enabling the practitioner to assess the overall picture and to perceive the problem from another angle. These views may or may not agree with the client's, but will allow the practitioner to observe family interactions and to bear these in mind when considering how to intervene. When carrying out an assessment, the practitioner uses counselling and relationship-building skills that facilitate an atmosphere of trust where the client feels it safe to reveal their concerns and feelings. It may not always be possible for practitioners to have all their questions answered due to clients having their own agenda. The client may have a particular issue they want to discuss and could be frustrated by any attempt to divert them from this. If the practitioner is successful in establishing a safe environment the client may take the opportunity to 'abreact'. Practitioners will then find themselves having to manage and facilitate healthy emotional catharsis as the client vents anger, frustration, or guilt, and displays acute distress. These times can be very therapeutic and should not be averted by the practitioner insisting on getting back to history taking. The assessment may require another session, or even be ongoing, with an initial report being sent to the referrer.

One of the aims of a first visit will be to assess the appropriateness of the referral. By the end of the visit the practitioner will either have decided that this is an appropriate referral for their discipline and that they have the knowledge and level of skill to take on the case, or that the client's needs can better be met by referring on to a colleague or another discipline. Although the first visit is for initial assessment, a therapeutic rapport or even therapy can commence when the practitioner is successful in gaining the client's confidence and trust.

The following list summarizes aims that practitioners could use when making both initial and subsequent home visits.

1. **Introduction** – explaining professional role and stating the purpose of the visit.
2. **Assessment** – gaining the client's and the family/carer's view of the problem.
3. **Appropriateness** – determining if the referral is within the practitioner's remit and whether they have the skills to meet the client's needs.
4. **Rapport** – the use of relationship-building skills to enhance the assessment and plan intervention.
5. **Care plan** – obtaining the client's agreement on the problem areas, and the action to be taken to resolve these.
6. **Contract** – the practitioner, in partnership with the client, agrees goals, frequency of sessions and review dates.

ALERTS AND EMERGENCIES (*see also* Anxiety management; Relaxation techniques; Coping and violence)

Although the majority of interactions are foreseen, there are times when prompt action is needed by the practitioner. These include the following situations.

Extrapyramidal side effects

Many of the neuroleptic drugs used in treatments produce side effects which are similar to Parkinsonism. They may come on extremely suddenly and are distressing to the client, needing prompt action. Examples of these are shaking, restlessness, tremor and stiffness of the limbs. In extreme cases an oculogyric crisis occurs, where the eyeballs rotate right up and the head tips back. Where any of these symptoms are seen, it is important that the client's GP is alerted as soon as possible so that an intramuscular injection of Procyclidine can be given to relieve the symptoms.

Panic attacks

This is a period of intense anxiety or fear which may last from minutes to hours. During this time the client may experience any of the following: chest pains, palpitations, choking or smothering feelings, dizziness, nausea, tingling in the hands or feet, hot and cold flushes, shaking and hyperventilating. The client needs immediate reassurance and practical measures should be taken to reduce the severity of their symptoms. Clients are scared that their symptoms are life threatening, particularly when these affect breathing or heart rate. The practitioner therefore should stay with them, letting the client know of their continued presence, until the symptoms begin to reduce. Hyperventilation is particularly frightening for the client, since the overbreathing caused by panic or fear inevitably leads to more anxiety. Breathing into cupped hands or into a paper bag will increase the amount of carbon dioxide and stabilize levels of both that and oxygen, so that breathing will slow down. Loosening any tight clothing and decreasing environmental stimuli such as excessive noise and bright lights will also help to reduce anxiety. In the longer term, help should be offered on anxiety reduction.

Aggression

Clients' non-verbal and verbal behaviour should be carefully noted since this alerts to the possibility of aggression occurring, for example restlessness, staring or repetitive movements. Should there be any hint that the client is becoming aggressive, practitioners should attempt to position themselves between the client and the door, so that an exit can be made as quickly as possible. If, however, injury results, immediate advice must be received from the manager as to the procedures to be followed.

Overdose

This may be accidental or non-accidental, but the immediate procedures to be followed are the same. It is helpful if it can be ascertained what the client has taken by observation of the area, checking pockets or asking significant others who are present, since if the client needs admission to hospital the more information that arrives with them the better. For specific presentations, consult *The British National Formulary*.

Lithium, acute toxic effects

Most cases arise as a result of long term lithium therapy, where the drug is excreted in reduced amounts. Presentation of this may be slight at first, with slight restlessness; but if this continues, vomiting, weakness and tremor occur. It is important to ensure that the next dose is not taken until a doctor has been consulted and a blood test for lithium levels has been taken.

ANXIETY MANAGEMENT (*see also* Relaxation techniques)

The client who suffers from unrealistic or excessive worry about life circumstances may experience a wide variety of physical and emotional effects. The overall feeling is of being unwell although specific complaints include gastrointestinal symptoms such as pain, nausea and vomiting, fatigue, palpitations, sweating and frequent urination. Any body system is likely to be involved; this can add to the client's anxiety, as they fear that something is seriously wrong with them. There is often an inability to concentrate, problems sleeping and changes in eating habits. Attempts to reduce the anxiety may lead to the over-use of addictive substances such as alcohol or tranquillizers, or the development of compulsive behaviours. The client is generally worried about themselves and about the loss of control over their lives. A particular difficulty for the client suffering from anxiety is feeling ashamed of their illness; in addition, they worry about the effects that it may have on other members of the family.

Treatments for anxiety are many faceted and challenging both for the practitioner and the client. The relationship between the two is crucial to the success of the methods used, since the client needs to feel safe to discuss matters of which they may feel ashamed and also to try new behaviours which involve some risk. The building of an empathic, warm relationship is obviously the first step and cannot be hurried without the client feeling that they are a nuisance.

A first step in the management of anxiety is to encourage the client to become fully aware of the anxiety in their lives. This may be achieved by asking the client to keep a daily journal to include a record of their feelings, anxieties, stressors and any precipitating factors with a note of the effects that any of these have on their physical or emotional well being. The rationale behind this is that the client can begin to make the mental link between feelings that they experience and the possible causes for them. Included in this daily account may be some way of rating the severity of their feelings, for example on a scale of one to ten, accompanying this with the times of day when the symptoms are present. From this a picture begins to emerge of the pattern of the anxiety, enabling more detailed care to be planned. The diary will also give the client a clearer picture of what may be causing the anxiety. Identifying the pattern of the anxiety and the possible causes helps the client to feel more in control and also optimistic about the treatment that they may need. Discussing their life style is useful to build up a picture of what is a realistic treatment plan for the client, as there is no point in recommending a treatment which is incompatible with this.

Treatment involves a combination of approaches. The listening, counselling approach enables the client to explore the stressors and feelings that they have identified and gives them the opportunity to understand, in a safe and supportive relationship, the effects of these on their emotions and daily life. Many GP surgeries now 'prescribe' exercise vouchers that can be redeemed at the local sports centre and clients often discover that regular physical exercise is an effective means of decreasing the physical effects of anxiety. This can be encouraged by the practitioner in ways ranging from a gentle walk every day to strenuous aerobic activity. Role playing will give the client an opportunity to explore new behaviours and new coping strategies. Education about diet may be appropriate, particularly for the client who is abusing stimulants. (The daily journal will have identified problem areas such as overeating or substance abuse.) Relaxation techniques can also be successful in overcoming the continual feelings of tension that can make life quite unbearable for the client.

APPOINTMENTS (*see also* Referral process)

In response to a referral, the practitioner will need to arrange for the first assessment meeting to take place. If the practitioner has been introduced to the referred client in the setting of a hospital ward or outpatient clinic, then this appointment will probably be arranged verbally.

If the referral has been received by telephone or letter, then appointments are made according to local policy. These procedures will vary from team to team, but in the main the practitioner will need to consider the following questions.

1. Is the client referred aware that the referral has been made?
2. Is the referrer aware of the referral's receipt and allocation?
3. Is it planned that the first contact will take place in the client's home, in the practitioner's territory such as a base or clinic, or in some other, neutral, environment?
4. Will the first appointment be arranged by telephone or by letter?

Telephone appointments are usually acceptable when an urgent response to the referral is required. Telephone appointments are also often used for arranging subsequent appointments not arranged at the time of the last meeting.

However, where possible, a letter is the preferred method of initial contact as it enables the client to check the authenticity of the communication and ensures that their case notes have recorded confirmation of the planned contact for initial assessment.

This letter to the client should, ideally, communicate the following information.

1. **How** the practitioner came to know of the client, that is name the referrer.
2. **Why** the referral to the practitioner has been made, that is for help, support, assessment or treatment.
3. **Where** the planned venue is to be, that is client's home, practitioner's base or clinic.
4. **When** the appointment is to take place, that is time and date.
5. **What** can the client do to change the appointment time or venue, or to seek further information, that is the practitioner's telephone number and the team's title and address.

The referrer could then be informed of the date of the first meeting by telephone or by receiving a copy of the appointment letter to the client.

ASSESSMENT (*see also* Observation and monitoring)

Ward (1985) defines assessment as 'the measurement of the patient's ability to function independently and the comparison of that ability with the level of behaviour he must achieve to bring about true self sufficiency'. Obtaining a full picture of the life of the client will therefore result in a practitioner being able to identify the client's needs and what he can and cannot achieve for himself.

However, while this process in an institutional setting is made easier by 24-hour observation and monitoring, a different approach obviously has to be adopted in community mental health care. If the client is being discharged from hospital into the community, then good liaison work beforehand with the hospital nursing staff will ensure continuity of care.

The community practitioner can have access to all the nursing records kept while the client has been in hospital. This means that they can see a record of the care that has been given, gain an overview of the needs of the client while in hospital and then use this knowledge as a basis for assessing the client's future needs after discharge. In the case of a new referral to the community team, where there is no previous knowledge of the client, thorough assessment is obtained from wider sources of information. The practitioner, not having the benefit of 24-hour observation, must rely not only on observations and problem identification from the client but also from as many people as possible with whom the client comes into contact. Starting with the immediate family, this radiates out to friends and neighbours if relevant, and to any other health professionals who may be involved. Information gathered in this way slowly forms a whole picture of the life of the client.

The client living in the community, as far as possible, is aiming to maintain as independent a life style as possible. The assessment, therefore, will focus on what this means, what is hindering its achievement and the physical, environmental and emotional resources the client and practitioner between them can utilize. The involvement of the client is crucial in the assessment process, since it is this independent life style, and not an adherence to institutional styles, that is being aimed for.

Basic data to be addressed include areas such as the level of independence of the client, how the client perceives the problem, how relevant carers perceive it, and the client's and carers' goals for the future.

Most community mental health teams will have their own assessment profile forms, giving a pro forma for guidance. If these are shown to the client, it will help to reassure and inform that this gathering of information, which may seem excessive sometimes, is the best way to plan care on a needs-driven basis. Prioritizing these identified needs is then possible with the client. It may be that the client and practitioner do not agree on these, and compromise may be needed, or to rethink alternatives. Once the priorities have been identified, it may then be possible also to identify needs that are less important, but which are still hindering the client's life style. The assessment is therefore always a joint production, with the client involved as much as possible, so that the impression is not given of a process in which the client is a passive participant. This is vital, as the practitioner will not be with the client all the time during the next stages of the nursing process: if the client has played an active part in the assessment process it will help to ensure their willingness to make further plans and to be involved in carrying them out.

Obviously, during the assessment, the level of risk to the patient is a priority. Actual or imminent life threatening concerns must be assessed; for example is the client expressing ideas such as 'I ought to be dead', which demonstrates a high level of suicidal ideation or a total disregard for personal safety. Here, observation of the congruence between verbal and non-verbal communication is crucial, since the client wishing to conceal such feelings may still reveal them non-verbally. Once life threatening concerns have been assessed, then actual or potential health threatening concerns should also be assessed. There are many assessment tools which can be used here, such as the *Beck Inventory for Measuring Depression* (Beck *et al.*, 1961), where the client chooses a series of statements that fit most closely to their present emotional state. One set of statements, for example, ranges in level of feelings about oneself from 'I don't feel disappointed in myself' to 'I do feel disappointed in myself'. The client and practitioner, by walking through these together, can clarify the state of mind of the client where previously he or she may have been unable to verbalize this. The client may also be encouraged to keep a day-to-day diary, which contributes to the assessment, in which questions such as 'what happened today?', and 'how did you feel about that?' can be answered. It has been stressed that the client must be fully involved in determining the priority of concerns and in considering the range of resources that are or could become available as they help implement the treatment plan that will be formulated as a result of such thorough assessment.

B

BEHAVIOURAL PSYCHOTHERAPY

Mental health nurses have been practising behavioural psychotherapy since the 1970s in a role that has come to be known as the behavioural nurse therapist. In the 1960s there was general dissatisfaction with psychoanalysis, which sparked interest in the development of alternative therapies. Behavioural approaches have been found to be beneficial in the treatment of obsessional compulsive disorder and were developed to treat a variety of other anxiety disorders. As the approach grew in popularity and efficacy there arose a shortage of skilled health professionals to meet the growing demand for treatment.

In the early 1970s Isaac Marks, a psychiatrist at the Institute of Psychiatry in London, advocated that mental health nurses be trained to become primary therapists. This was highly controversial at the time as many psychiatrists and psychologists argued that mental health nurses did not possess the required degree of clinical sophistication to operate as independent therapists. In addition it is now acknowledged that a number of these professionals felt that their skills monopoly was under threat. However, despite the opposition a pilot scheme was set up to train nurses as behavioural therapists and they were found to treat patients as effectively as other clinicians within the field. Since the 1970s nurses have continued to be trained and now practice behavioural psychotherapy and cognitive behaviour therapy in the treatment of a wide variety of mental health problems and in a wide variety of different settings.

Until the 1970s behavioural psychotherapy derived its main theoretical basis from experiential psychology. Since then it has developed into a discipline which has weathered criticisms and continues to evolve and innovate in clinical practice. Behavioural psychotherapy comprises a range of therapeutic methods which change abnormal behaviour directly rather than by analysing hypothesized interpersonal conflicts. The presenting problem could be a behavioural deficit such as phobic avoidance or a behavioural excess such as compulsive rituals which cause distress.

The main principles of therapy are that it is problem-orientated, structured, active, empirically based, time-limited, collaborative and founded on research-based psychological methods. The aim of treatment is to alter the behaviour that restricts the patient's social, work and day-to-day life. The main disorders treated are phobic disorders, obsessive compulsive disorder, sexual dysfunction, alternative sexual practices, habit disorders, eating disorders, anger management, stress management and habit disorders.

Cognitive behaviour therapy draws on the theories of cognitive therapy, especially those of Beck and Emery (Beck and Emery, 1985). It incorporates these theories with behavioural approaches and techniques. Cognitive behaviour therapy is used in the treatment of depression, post-traumatic stress disorder, hypochondriasis, chronic fatigue and generalized anxiety disorder.

Nurse therapists work as autonomous practitioners who manage their individual caseloads, assess, treat, evaluate and discharge patients whom they have found suitable for treatment. As clinical specialists there is usually an advisory and consultancy element to their work coupled with supervisory, training and educative roles. Nurse therapists are often freed from the operational constraints to which other nurses are routinely subjected such as manpower planning and on call duties. This facilitates reflective practice and professional independence. Currently work and research is growing in the use of cognitive behavioural therapy with individuals suffering long and enduring mental illness such as schizophrenia.

BEREAVEMENT

Most of us can expect to experience the loss of a loved one at some stage during our lives. Most individuals go through the grieving process and eventually adjust to the loss with the help and support of their family and friends. Others may obtain additional support and counselling from such organizations as Cruse or the Samaritans.

Most individuals proceed through their grief in a healthy way that facilitates acceptance, adaptation and a fresh identity. Bereavement is one of the major life events and involves challenge and readjustment.

Unhealthy forms of grief are sometimes called morbid, atypical or abnormal grief reactions, and the bereaved person may present as ill. Pathological processes of the illness can be seen as intensifications, deviations or prolongations of processes that occur in health (Bowlby, 1980). Referrals will generally only come to mental health practitioners when the referrer suspects evidence of a pathological component in the grief process. This pathology might display as overt anxiety or panic attacks, clinical depression, suicidal ideas, inappropriate rituals or the inability to move forward in the process of mourning. Colin Murray Parkes's (1972) studies of grief enabled him to describe the nature of the principal components of the reaction to bereavement. These components complemented the stages described in John Bowlby's work in the 1980s. When the components are called stages it can mistakenly give the impression that all the components have to be gone through, and in the correct order, before acceptance and adjustment can be achieved. However, it is possible for a component to be absent or for an individual to experience a return to an earlier component.

Ramsey (1979) lists nine components of griefwork that professionals can recognize.

1. **Shock** – this is the physical reaction experienced as numbness and disbelief. The physiological changes associated with shock are displayed.
2. **Disorganization** – the individual's routine is broken. There may be confusion or bewilderment as former ways of coping seem invalidated. Family and friends temporarily take over some tasks.
3. **Denial** – there may be attempts to postpone the reality of the loss. The individual may state that the loss has not happened, or that the loved one will appear. There may be attempts to continue with routines that are now redundant due to the loss. Alcohol may be used to anaesthetize painful feelings and the reality of the loss.
4. **Depression** – this may present as non-clinical with the expression of crying and great sadness or as a clinical depression with freezing of affect, self-neglect, withdrawal from reality and suicidal thoughts.
5. **Guilt** – this component usually involves issues of self-blame, that is 'If only I had …' There is often a preoccupation with the events leading up to the death of the loved one.
6. **Anxiety** – this can present as loss of confidence and insecurity. Pining and searching behaviour may take place. In this component, the individual may fall into a helpless role.
7. **Aggression** – the individual bereaved may focus blame and anger onto self, family, doctors, God or even the deceased. Answers as to 'why' may be sought.
8. **Resolution** – during this component there is a 'psychological burial'. The individual accepts that the loved one is not coming back, and change at a cognitive level takes place.
9. **Acceptance** – the individual accepts that 'life goes on' and is able to move forward and commence a new routine. The practitioner will recognize the components and reassure the bereaved person that the experience is natural and that fears of going mad are unfounded.

During bereavement counselling the practitioner facilitates the expression of grief, to 'give sorrow words', rather than keep feelings bottled up. The bereaved often complain that well-meaning family and friends avoid talking about the deceased. Trivial conversation and the avoidance of overt emotion tends to reduce the value of the loss in the mind of the bereaved. It can be a great relief to the bereaved person when they are given 'permission' to grieve. If any unhealthy processes are observed, the practitioner is able either to work directly with the client on these problems or refer on to a psychologist or psychiatrist as appropriate.

BOUNDARY SETTING

Within the practitioner–client relationship the setting and maintenance of boundaries is of utmost importance. Boundary setting enables the relationship to function within a framework in which both parties are aware of individual roles, limitations and expectations. At the outset of the relationship the practitioner and client should discuss what their expectations and needs are from the relationship. These may include:

- **how?** – both parties should be able to access the meeting place easily;
- **what?** – both parties should be aware of what they are meeting for and the purpose of the meetings;
- **why?** – both parties should be aware of why they are meeting, the length of time, period of time between meetings and whether it is expected that the relationship will be short or long term;
- **when?** – both parties should be aware of when they are meeting.

The boundary setting should not be dictated by either party but negotiated to ensure that each person is able to achieve their goals.

Professional boundaries

The professional boundaries that exist for the practitioner and client involve the fact that the practitioner is seen as the person with expert knowledge within the relationship. It must be remembered that the client is the person with the most knowledge of their particular mental health problems and the circumstances surrounding them. The practitioner may be seen as an authority figure of higher status and this creates an unequal relationship with the practitioner in a position of power. Although little can be done to change this it is important that the practitioner is aware of the effect of their role on the relationship. Often the relationship between practitioner and client can develop and become what appears to be one of friendship and may be regarded as such by those involved. Both parties need to be aware that this is not the case as the practitioner has a professional duty to the client to maintain a therapeutic relationship in which they administer care, either physical, therapeutic or both. As the practitioner may be the only person to whom the client can relate, trust or confide they may regard the relationship as more than a professional one. Practitioners should be sure of their professional boundaries and ensure that clients are aware of them.

CARE PROGRAMME APPROACH (CPA)

Since 1st April 1991 all specialist mental health services have been required to formalize aftercare following inpatient treatment and community care for all clients referred to them in the form of care programmes. The care programmes should describe the health care needs of the client and the services which would be provided to assist the person to maintain optimum health in the community. The requirements of the Care Programme Approach (CPA) were first described in the Department of Health circular HC (DoH, 1990). In addition to the programme describing the client's needs and the care to be provided the CPA also requires that each patient has a designated keyworker who will be responsible for coordinating the delivery of care described in the care programme.

Implementation of the CPA has been problematic since its introduction, which is probably due to the degree of flexibility and interpretation in the initial documentation. CPA is exactly what it is titled, an approach rather than a prescription. It does no more than describe in broad principles what was previously best practice in community mental health services. That is, people with mental health problems in the community receiving care from trained mental health professionals (predominantly mental health nurses), the care provided being systematically recorded and evaluated with regular multidisciplinary or multi-agency reviews as appropriate.

Another major difficulty in implementation of CPA has been definition of the client group, combined with a perception that a huge new volume of work has been created at a stroke. The intended client group is people with serious and enduring mental health problems; unfortunately there is no agreed definition of what constitutes a serious and enduring mental illness.

The Department of Health publication *Building Bridges, A guide to arrangements for interagency working for the care and protection of severely mentally ill people* (DoH, 1995a) seeks to provide a framework around which services can agree a local working definition. They suggest five dimensions for the definition and these are:

- disability
- diagnosis
- duration
- safety
- the need for informal or formal care.

The problem created by the perception of the volume of new work has been addressed in the second edition of the *Mental Illness Key Areas Handbook* (DoH, 1994c). Chapter 9 of this publication introduces the concept of tiered CPA.

> The requirement that the CPA apply to all patients in contact with specialist psychiatric services does not mean that the multidisciplinary team will need to be involved with every patient. There are in fact several possible levels of CPA, depending of the severity of the patient's condition. Services should apply the requirements of the CPA sensitively, to ensure the full multidisciplinary CPA is applied only to those patients who need it. Although other patients who are in contact with specialist services should still receive the basic help of the CPA, they will not need the same input of staff time.

> A model of tiered CPA is described at some length in Appendix 9.3 of the *Key Areas Handbook*. The most common model currently in use has three tiers: the lowest is minimal CPA where a single mental health professional is responsible for the care programme, for example, a community mental health nurse managing the client's care independently with routine reporting to the multidisciplinary team at agreed review dates. The second tier is more complex, with more than one member of the multidisciplinary team being involved but usually only one agency being involved in the delivery of care, for example, services from the mental health trust. The third tier, or full multidisciplinary CPA as it is known in some areas, involves care delivered by more than one member of the multidisciplinary team and more than one agency, for example, the mental health trust and the social services department.

> The most significant factor of the tiered approach for community mental health nurses is the range of roles that they may play in different tiers. As stated previously, within the minimal CPA the community mental health nurse will normally be the nominated keyworker, responsible for the production, delivery and evaluation of the care programme. At the next level the community mental health nurse may well still be the nominated

keyworker but will have the additional responsibility of co-ordinating the delivery of other elements of the care programme which he or she does not deliver directly. In the most complex care programmes the community mental health nurse may be either the nominated keyworker or may deliver a component of a care programme for which another member of the team is the nominated keyworker.

Keyworker responsibilities in complex care programmes have an additional, time consuming, administrative responsibility which requires both training and allocated time. The responsibilities of keyworking need to be agreed locally, particularly between health and social services departments who are the most common partners in the delivery of complex care programmes. An agreement should lead to formal training sessions for all members of the multidisciplinary team. This should lead to consistency in the recording and delivery of care programmes on a basis of shared understanding of local protocols and documentation. The NHS Training Division has published a strategic development pack to support the progression of local CPA implementation entitled *Building on Strengths* (NHS, 1995). This contains both valuable information about the CPA and straightforward training exercises which can be used locally.

The CPA, when properly implemented, inevitably leads to more paperwork than was the case before April 1991. However, the benefits of a properly formulated, recorded and managed care programme in association with the designated keyworker are irrefutable. These benefits can only be maximized in an environment where staff are properly trained in the requirements of the CPA and sufficient time is allocated to the keyworkers of complex care programmes to carry out their coordinating responsibilities as well as their care responsibilities.

CARERS (*see also* Stress and coping)

The role of the carer has received increasing attention in the past few years, with recognition of the demands placed on them by the client in the community. Family members may feel that they have, in some way, contributed to the problems faced by the client and this can lead to an over compensation in their care resulting in fatigue and depression. This is particularly common in the care of the elderly where the physical and emotional demands on the carers can be very high. The carer may become easily irritable and shout at the person for whom they are caring, resulting in feelings of guilt. In some cases, the individual may provoke hostility and receive physical abuse as a result of a break in the carer's tolerance. The act of caring for someone with any type of mental illness may have several effects on the carer such as a reduction in income, disruption to the social and domestic life of the family, and problems of ill health caused by the pressures (Simmons and Morrisey, 1995). Some carers are unaware, for example, that they are entitled to extra benefits such as Attendance Allowance and advice in this direction can help to take some of the pressure off the family. The role of the practitioner as a health educator is to be emphasized here. Where information can be given to the carers about, for example, the illness itself, what behaviours can be expected and how they can be treated, this will help to reduce their anxiety. Membership of support groups can be suggested, and the addresses of resources given so that carers are able to get help with any of the problems that can arise, whether these are emotional, social or environmental. Practical services and aids may need to be supplemented by counselling support to enable them to continue to bear the burden of caring or reach the point where others take over part or the whole of their responsibilities. By providing this support, the carers can be helped to express their frustrations and anxieties without fear of being judged or seen as failures. Carers often express feelings of being trapped and of having no life of their own. These feelings may be kept hidden so as not to appear selfish and it may be a great relief to be able to verbalize them. Simmons (1984) conducted a study into family carers and concluded that the practitioner has a vital role in working with the carers as well as with the client, in order that they can feel a sense of value and that the importance of their role is recognized. This involvement of the carers at all stages of the nursing process will also be of benefit to the practitioner who can use the resources and skills that they have in order to ensure continuity of care for the client and the maximum use of resources.

CASE MANAGEMENT

Case management is defined by Onyett (1994) as involving 'assessing and meeting users' needs rather than managing service provision'. This differs from the term 'care management' which applies to the management of case management and provider agencies at a higher management tier (Challis, 1990). Case management is the provision of help specifically designed to meet a client's requirements through the assessment and service coordination undertaken by one individual worker or team. Onyett (1994) describes the core tasks of being a case manager as follows.

1. **Assessment** – clarification of a client's needs and strengths.
2. **Planning** – the development of a plan with clear specific outcomes, easily understood.
3. **Implementation** – with the involvement of users, their relevant supporters and a chosen range of agencies to meet the various needs identified.
4. **Monitoring** – progress, and/or lack of progress towards the specified objectives is systematically monitored and recorded.
5. **Reviewing** – outcomes of the planned interventions are evaluated with all those involved in the work. This may take the form of reassessment and introduce a restart of the cycle.

There are different models of case management and in some cases case managers may act as therapist, counsellor, advocate or broker for other helping agencies, involving the purchasing of services.

'Case management can increase the flexibility, continuity and responsiveness of mental health service provision by assigning clear responsibilities to individual staff working within teams' (Onyett, 1994). It is becoming more prevalent within community mental health care teams and the concepts and ideology of this model needs to be understood. Further reading is recommended.

CLINICAL AUDIT

Clinical audit can be defined as 'the systematic and critical analysis of the quality of care, including the procedures used for diagnosis, treatment and care; the associated use of resources and the resulting outcome and quality of life for the patient' (DOH, 1993b). Clinical audit can be stated as a systematic review and improvement in the delivery of care to the patient. The Department of Health recommends that the principles should:

• be led by clinical professionals;
• involve the views of patients;
• form a part of routine clinical practice;
• be an educational process;
• involve management in the process and outcomes;
• generate results that are used to improve quality of care.

To be able to perform audit it is necessary to have time, commitment and understanding. It is an excellent opportunity for all members of the client care team to generate evidence to improve the quality of care.

Audit differs from research in that it seeks to examine whether actual practice matches the standards set. Research involves investigation and the generation or testing of a theory.

Audit cycle

The audit cycle comprises three main stages:

1. defining the expected level of quality;
2. measuring and comparing practice against the expected level;
3. action plan for improvement.

When defining the expected level of quality it is necessary to identify the audit topic, agreeing a standard, formulating criteria and implementing the standard. The measurement and comparison stage involves actual practice being compared against the criteria defined in the standard. It is important to select the most appropriate methods of data collection; this may be retrospective and should combine the gathering of information from different sources (clients, practitioners, carers, documentation) and the use of a range of methods (interviewing, observation, questionnaire). The sample size for the audit exercise needs to be identified and should reflect a representation of what happens in the practice area. The action plan is necessary for change and improvement to occur.

Successful audit depends upon client involvement, team work and organizational support.

CLINICAL SUPERVISION (*see also* Management supervision; Setting up supervision)

Since Vision for the Future, the Allitt Enquiry and Strategy for Nursing, clinical supervision has become high on the agenda of professional nursing issues. Community mental health care has been more fortunate than most areas of nursing as for many clinical supervision has been an accepted integral part of working life. The need for clinical supervision is resisted by some and welcomed by many; that it is a directive from the Department of Health enables health care organizations to ensure that practitioners have access to clinical supervision.

There are a number of definitions and interpretations of clinical supervision.

- Clinical supervision is about a relationship between two or more people.
- The relationship is a professional one.
- Each person has a specific role within the relationship, either supervisee or supervisor.
- The relationship is a confidential one.
- The process of supervision is a facilitative one where the supervisee is enabled to examine their practice in a supportive environment.
- The supervisor should not tell the supervisee what to do but challenge and inform in a constructive manner.

All these issues appear to be clear to most practitioners but from examining projects and literature regarding the implementation of clinical supervision it is apparent that many organizations have little understanding of the process of supervision. Often practitioners perceive supervision as an appraisal, observation of clinical work, managerial and disciplinary in nature. It may be that many practitioners feel more comfortable with this format as it involves tasks and behaviours. Clinical supervision involves the effective domain and it is this area with which practitioners historically have most difficulty (Menzies, 1960).

The process of clinical supervision involves exploring issues arising from a practitioner's area of work; the focus of these may be caseload, educational, professional or practice development. Often the content of the supervision session will overlap all of these areas. Supervision should enable the examination of affective, conative and cognitive approaches to an area of practice. Normative, formative and restorative functions as described by Proctor (1986) should be allowed to occur. The supervisor is akin to a leader, encouraging the supervisee to examine practice and explore the way forward, whether these be resolutions, new developments, the need to gain skills or develop academically. To achieve this the supervisor requires extensive skills in facilitation, challenging and guidance. Expertise in the relevant area practice of the supervisee is debatable. Some believe that the supervisor should be a clinical expert in a specialist area and only supervise practitioners in that area: the skills of supervision, however, lie in the process of enablement. If a supervisor has both qualities, then fine but there is no reason why a supervisor who is not from the same specialist area of practice cannot offer effective supervision. It is the supervisee's responsibility to seek information, additional expert clinical knowledge where appropriate and applicable training to develop areas of development identified in supervision sessions.

The supervisor is objective – able to stand outside the issues raised, to see clearly, to seek to enable clarification and to allow the supervisee to view the issues more ably (in other words, to distinguish the wood from the trees).

The supervisee requires skills: skills to negotiate their supervision time, skills to use this time most effectively and skills to write up their sessions enabling further reflection on the supervision.

Training for both supervisor and supervisee to develop the skills required for the most effective supervision is recommended (Butterworth, 1994; Kohner, 1994).

CLOSURES

It is often quite difficult when in a client's home, their territory, to close a session. The end of an interaction can have a clear effect on the next encounter with the client. For example, after a session in which a lot of emotion has been expressed, it is important not to end the interaction too abruptly so that the client does not feel that all the release of emotion has been unrecognized and unacknowledged. In this instance, the practitioner can positively reinforce the honesty of the client and the cost of such expression of feeling. At the same time, to allow the closure to extend for too long may result in too much dependency on the practitioner. Time pressures may mean that, even subtly, the client feels that he or she is being hurried, and that therefore he or she is not important. However, there are times when the client will try to prolong the ending of a session, because of wanting more input, needing more reassurance or being lonely and wanting company. However this appeal to stay makes the practitioner feel the contractual agreement normally entered into must be honoured by saying, for example 'we did agree that our sessions would last for an hour, which is now over. As you know, though, I will be back on Thursday, and we can carry on discussing this then'. Both client and practitioner need to have equal opportunity for closure, to reinforce what has been achieved, and to end with the recognition of the bond that has been maintained in the session. Closing on a positive note will give the client this sense of achievement. For example, practitioners can preface the meeting arrangements for the following session by saying something like 'I feel that a lot of useful work has been done today, and I look forward to seeing you again next week'.

COMMUNICATION AND RELATIONSHIP-BUILDING TECHNIQUES – DIFFERENT APPROACHES TO THE THERAPEUTIC RELATIONSHIP (*see also* Drama techniques)

Communication and relationship-building skill difficulties may be areas with which clients possess lifelong problems. There are a number of different media apart from verbal skills that may be used to allow for the ventilation of feelings, relating of experiences and development of the relationship between mental health nurse and client.

These media include the use of clay, paints, writing or story-telling. Clay enables the diversion of thoughts into creating pieces of work through which expression of emotion may be made, along with the sense of achievement gained by the production of a work of art. Painting and drawing enables the expressions of feelings (well demonstrated by artists such as Van Gogh). The practitioner's role is to work with the client in sharing the drawing or painting (particularly effective for clients who are mute or withdrawn or experiencing long-term illness through which their relationship-building skills are diminished). It is not the practitioner's role to interpret the painting but to offer the client the chance to describe in their own words what they have painted. The practitioner should ask questions sensitively to enable the client to open up.

Story-telling involves the client writing their own story or the practitioner writing it verbatim whilst the client speaks and then giving it to the client to check. Alternatively a diary may be maintained by the client who then reads out selected parts. It is often easier for the client to talk about their feelings by reading a script, the script being theirs. This enables clients who feel unable to put their feelings into words orally to confront them when expressed on paper. Many of these activities are offered in day hospitals or resource centres but a large number of clients are unable to attend for a variety of reasons. It is important therefore that the community mental health nurses avail themselves of a variety of tools to enable the development and use of communication and relationship-building skills.

CONFIDENTIALITY (*see also* Access to Health Records Act (1990); Data Protection Act 1984)

The client entering a therapeutic relationship will inevitably have concerns about the amount of information that will be passed to the practitioner and how that information will be stored and used. On the initial meeting and whenever necessary after that, the practitioner needs to explain clearly what is understood by confidentiality. The client should understand that by this it is meant that any information passed to the practitioner remains there with certain provisos. If the practitioner is part of a larger team, then the client must be told that if it helps the team to provide better care for the client, then information may be passed on to them. Similarly, the practitioner must report behaviour that has or may occur which could be dangerous. This is, however, a difficult judgement to make and the practitioner should seek guidance from the appropriate manager before releasing such information. Giving information to the client about confidentiality helps to reassure them about revealing personal material; it also means that the client and practitioner are able to review the boundaries of their relationship. It is important that the client is aware that he or she has the right **not** to disclose information, and the right therefore to privacy. This knowledge ensures that the client is able to maintain control, and does not have to feel pumped for information.

The practitioner must also be aware that the client can now request to see medical records, and this may influence record keeping to avoid making value judgements on what is known about the client.

COPING AND VIOLENCE (*see also* Diffusing anger; Alerts and emergencies)

Students coming into mental health practice often express concern about the likelihood of encountering violence. Research such as Whittington and Wykes (1994) indicates that the violence that occurs tends to be more in the nature of verbal abuse, and that the incidence of physical injury is low (HSAC, 1987). However, the experience of being exposed to abuse of any type can be traumatic for any practitioner and it is important, therefore, to be aware of the likelihood of it occurring and strategies for coping with it.

Verbal abuse such as racist and sexist remarks or verbal intimidation of any kind can sap the confidence of the recipient, often resulting in them feeling very vulnerable. While the violence, whether physical or verbal, is occurring the recipient is having to make a rapid assessment of the situation. For example, would any approach made now make a difference to the situation; could the situation be defused; should I remove myself from the area now and so on. Confrontation might allow for the facilitation of the client's feelings, but this is hard to achieve successfully unless the client is well known to the practitioner. An assertive approach may control and limit the amount of violence and practising this with one's colleagues is useful.

Where verbal techniques have not worked, unless the practitioner has specialist training in breakaway techniques, the client should never be grappled with since this could merely cause injury to either the client or the practitioner. In these circumstances, the immediate necessity is to get out of the area as quickly as possible, to raise the alarm and to get help, since the practitioner should never, in cases where the possibility of physical violence has become a reality, remain and attempt to tackle the problem alone.

It is important to explore one's feelings after the event, using a colleague for emotional support. Afterwards admitting to fear during the event, discussing feelings of weakness or self-blame for the event are all necessary to avoid future lack of confidence. The practitioner needs also to remember that the abuse, although directed at them, may not be related to them at all. The practitioner is merely in the situation when the client needs to release their own pain, and becomes the unwilling recipient of it. Discussing the event with a colleague also makes it a learning experience to think about how the situation could have been better handled. Practical measures, such as the possible need for a personal alarm and making sure that the team knows each person's whereabouts, are also ways in which the practitioner is able to feel more confident and supported by the team.

CRISIS INTERVENTION (*see also* Assessment; Alerts and emergencies)

Caplan (1961) sees the individual as living in a state of emotional equilibrium, which can easily be upset by major or minor threats; the more major the threat is perceived as by the individual, the greater the rise in emotional tension, leading, if unresolved, to a state of crisis. In this state, the individual's coping mechanisms are no longer adequate to cope with the feelings experienced at the time. These threats may occur as part of the developmental life of the individual, for example the menopause, or as unexpected life events, such as divorce or the loss of a job.

As a response to the crisis, the individual employs various strategies in an attempt to resolve the emergency and when these fail there is a resultant disorganization and disequilibrium. At this time the individual makes a clear appeal for help, verbally or non-verbally, which means that there is an ideal opportunity to move in quickly and become involved with the individual and his or her significant others. The principle of crisis intervention is to provide immediate, short-term help to restore the functioning of the individual.

The initial assessment is therefore most important. On meeting the client for the first time, it is important that the practitioner identifies exactly who they are, why they are there, and that they are taking the problem seriously.

They should find out from the client and their family if possible exactly what the problem is and how it has affected the client in every area of life. How have the family become aware of the crisis? What has been tried so far in an attempt to solve the problem and what happened as a result? What has been happening in the client's life during the last few days or weeks? While obtaining this information, the client's mental state should also be assessed: are there any suicidal thoughts apparent, how great is their distress or confusion? Once the practitioner feels that an accurate view of the situation has been obtained, he or she should feed this back to all involved in a way that demonstrates that the client's reactions are understandable. This is particularly important so that the individual does not feel ashamed at reacting in the way that they do, but can feel confident that the practitioner will work with them. Following this, the practitioner should explain very clearly the way in which he or she, the client and the family can work together on short-term goal planning and achievement. A crisis normally resolves within six weeks, so a contract for a few sessions can be offered, during which time a step by step approach to the crisis resolution is used. The client may feel quite ill with tiredness as a result of the emotional feelings that have been occurring, and restoration of a normal sleep pattern should be taken into account. Knowledge of resources available to offer extra support is invaluable, such as support groups and working with the client to increase self-esteem that was lost during the crisis. This is perhaps at the heart of crisis work, establishing a relationship that supports the client's normal view of themselves, and promoting adaptive behaviour to restore normal functioning as soon as possible.

CRISIS INTERVENTION TEAMS AND CRISIS RESPONSE TEAMS

The first of these was developed in the early 1970s at Napsbury Hospital, St Albans. Teams tend to be multiprofessional but in recent years uni-disciplinary response teams along with an on call service provision manned by community mental health nurses are becoming more popular. The purpose of these teams is to abate crisis in the client's home, either avoiding hospitalization and/or admitting the client to hospital with the intention of a short period of stay. They seek to meet the requirements of *The Patient's Charter* (DoH, 1995b) where urgent referrals from GPs are seen within two hours. As the models for these teams are variable it is useful to visit and examine the workings of teams already in place prior to setting up one's own response/intervention team.

They should find out from the client and their family if possible exactly what the problem is and how it has affected the client in every area of life. How have the family become aware of the crisis? What has been tried so far in an attempt to solve the problem and what happened as a result? What has been happening in the client's life during the last few days or weeks? While obtaining this information, the client's mental state should also be assessed: are there any suicidal thoughts apparent, how great is their distress or confusion? Once the practitioner feels that an accurate view of the situation has been obtained, he or she should feed this back to all involved in a way that demonstrates that the client's reactions are understandable. This is particularly important so that the individual does not feel ashamed at reacting in the way that they do, but can feel confident that the practitioner will work with them. Following this, the practitioner should explain very clearly the way in which he or she, the client and the family can work together on short-term goal planning and achievement. A crisis normally resolves within six weeks, so a contract for a few sessions can be offered, during which time a step by step approach to the crisis resolution is used. The client may feel quite ill with tiredness as a result of the emotional feelings that have been occurring, and restoration of a normal sleep pattern should be taken into account. Knowledge of resources available to offer extra support is invaluable, such as support groups and working with the client to increase self-esteem that was lost during the crisis. This is perhaps at the heart of crisis work, establishing a relationship that supports the client's normal view of themselves, and promoting adaptive behaviour to restore normal functioning as soon as possible.

CRISIS INTERVENTION TEAMS AND CRISIS RESPONSE TEAMS

The first of these was developed in the early 1970s at Napsbury Hospital, St Albans. Teams tend to be multiprofessional but in recent years uni-disciplinary response teams along with an on call service provision manned by community mental health nurses are becoming more popular. The purpose of these teams is to abate crisis in the client's home, either avoiding hospitalization and/or admitting the client to hospital with the intention of a short period of stay. They seek to meet the requirements of *The Patient's Charter* (DoH, 1995b) where urgent referrals from GPs are seen within two hours. As the models for these teams are variable it is useful to visit and examine the workings of teams already in place prior to setting up one's own response/intervention team.

D

DATA PROTECTION ACT 1984 (*see also* Confidentiality; Access to Health Records Act 1990)

This Act only applies to information about a client that is being held on computer. The underlying principles of the Act state that these records must be accurate, relevant, not kept longer than is necessary and not disclosed to unauthorized people. The person holding the information must be registered with the Data Protection Register, and anyone misusing the information is personally liable in law for that misuse. Under the terms of this Act, the client has the right to request to see their records although certain conditions are attached to this. Firstly, only a health professional can exercise the right of disclosure. Health professional is defined as either the medical practitioner who has overall care for the client or a registered nurse or similar. Secondly, there are two exemptions that apply to the disclosure of information. The first states that information cannot be disclosed if it is thought likely that exposure to the information could cause serious harm to the physical or mental health of the data subject and the second is that the information cannot be disclosed if such disclosure would reveal to the data subject the identity of another individual who has not consented to this information being seen. The client who wishes to exercise their rights under this Act applies to the holder of the computerized records, pays a fee and should be given the required information within 40 days, or told the grounds for withholding it. Any information disclosed that is inaccurate must be rectified and compensation may be paid for any harm that may have been suffered as a result of any inaccuracy.

DAY CARE FACILITIES

Closure of the large psychiatric hospitals has led to a need for the provision of day care facilities, not only for those with mild or moderate mental illness for whom a hospital bed was no longer felt to be appropriate, but also for the large numbers of those with a chronic mental illness who were discharged into the community from the large hospitals and who still needed support and monitoring of their condition. The provision of care varies nationally and is given by the health services, social services and voluntary and charitable bodies. However, the Audit Commission (1986) demonstrated that where hospital beds had been reduced by 25 500, day places had increased by only 9000. Day care provision centres varied between day hospitals and a range of day centres offering differing facilities according to the user group.

The focus of the day hospital is clearly treatment, and clients may be referred for sessional activities including one to one work or, depending on the severity of their condition, for attendance on a daily or weekly basis. The depot injection clinic is often centred at the day hospital, thus giving the team the opportunity to monitor and observe the client. Day hospitals, which normally are staffed by a full multidisciplinary team, including psychiatrists, nurses, social workers, occupational therapists and so on are able to provide a full range of therapeutic activities for clients such as social skills training, family therapy, assertiveness skills work and group therapy. They are normally open on weekdays only, although some do offer weekend facilities which meet the needs of the very vulnerable or isolated client.

With the reduction nationally in the numbers of hospital beds available, an increasing number of those with chronic mental health problems were discharged into the community with specific needs. Many of these clients live alone, often in bed and breakfast accommodation, and access to day care may be the only opportunity they have for social interactions or even for a meal shared with others. The emphasis of the day centre therefore focuses more on the need for supporting those who may have had years of institutional life and whose priorities will include learning how to live in the community. Day centres also often operate on a 'drop in' basis, thus catering for the needs of the homeless or the lonely; the day to day running of these centres is often provided by the users themselves who organize cooking, cleaning and other services.

Much has been written about the advantages and disadvantages of community care, often focussing on the lack of resources available for an ever-increasing client group. With the wide variety of resources available, however, it is essential that the practitioner has a thorough knowledge of the services available in the area, whether run by statutory or voluntary bodies, in order to enhance client care. Knowledge of local referral patterns is also important so that the client can take advantage of resources that will meet individual needs and not miss opportunities. With this knowledge, the client who is seen no longer to need, for example, the services provided by the day hospital can move to another centre without 'getting lost' and disappearing from sight. Liaison between all those working in day care facilities is therefore necessary, as is the need for flexible programmes that are tailored for the user group at the time. In many day care services, the use of the keyworker role is highlighted in meeting the needs of clients on an individual basis. This role is geared to coordinating and monitoring the care offered to clients, and acting as advocate in any sphere of the client's life if necessary, including liaising with essential services or providing information and support for carers.

DELUSIONS (*see also* Hallucinations; Disorientation)

Clare (1976) describes a delusion as 'not merely a false belief of morbid origin but an absolute conviction, not culturally shared, and is unamenable to reason, persuasion, contradiction or even the possibility of being in error. It is often preoccupying and usually absurd or impossible'. The term 'primary delusion' is used to describe the delusions experienced by a person who is suffering a schizophrenic illness. The experience can come without warning and may even puzzle the subject, yet the conviction persists. 'Secondary delusions' arise from some other morbid experience, for example, the nihilistic delusions seen in severe depression, or the grandiose delusions in mania. Acute confusional states caused by organic pathological processes including alcohol, drugs, infections and endocrine or neurological conditions may produce vague persecutory delusions alongside hallucinations and disorientation. These delusions abate once the underlying condition is treated. More persistent delusions occur in the disorders classified as the 'functional psychoses'. These include schizophrenia, affective psychosis and the paranoid disorders. These are mental disorders in which major disturbances of the mental processes may be seen (for instance hallucinations and delusions) but they differ from organic states in that they are not caused by any identified physical disease (Brooking *et al.*, 1992). These disturbances affect the individual's perception, thoughts and beliefs, and the delusions are often of a persecutory nature. In schizophrenia, the delusions include:

- delusional perception (where everyday events take on special significance for the client);
- passivity (the client believes and accepts control of his body by an external agent);
- thoughts that are either inserted, transmitted or stolen (Sugden *et al.*, 1986).

In the affective psychoses, the mood is disturbed and the individual may be elated (mania) or depressed (psychotic depression). In mania, grandiose delusions are common. In psychotic depression, delusions of guilt or worthlessness are usual, as are convictions of having cancer or some other serious illness or disease. Other delusions involve negative self-image. For example, clients may refuse to eat because they 'have no stomach'.

Delusions of persecution are common in the endogenous type of depression (though clients may accept them as justifiable punishment for wickedness) and clients frequently express delusions about their spouse being unfaithful or trying to poison them. If the delusion is depressive in origin then it should decrease in intensity or disappear as the depression subsides (Fottrell, 1983).

In depression, the delusions are in keeping with the content of the client's nihilistic ideas. The elderly, in particular, are likely to suffer from severe depression and often express delusions regarding perceived poverty, or guilt at having committed a sin or a crime. In young people, paranoia is usually indicative of schizophrenia but in the elderly it is very common and less serious. It is typically associated with solitary living, insecurity, anxiety and encounters with ageism (Brooking *et al.*, 1992).

Late paraphrenia is a term used for certain paranoid states of the elderly. This condition is more common in women and there is often associated sensory loss and social isolation. The delusions tend to have a rational basis and the individual tells of 'items going missing' or 'people breaking in'. Their delusions tend to be more localized in that the persecutory feelings are more likely to be attributed to a spouse, or, if living alone, a neighbour. In some cases, memory loss may contribute to misunderstanding and misinterpretation.

To treat delusions the practitioner will need to be skilful in establishing and maintaining a relationship and able to cope with rejection, hostility and unpredictable behaviour. The relationship will need to be developed gradually through regular contact, tolerance and perseverance. It can be a long process with frequent setbacks. The ability to communicate empathy and non-judgemental acceptance can help to establish rapport.

If the practitioner disagrees with the delusion then alienation can occur. If the practitioner agrees, then reinforcement will raise the client's anxiety level and therapy will be set back. One way of responding that can avoid this dilemma is to focus on the emotion underlying the belief. The belief may be false but the feelings of fear, insecurity or social alienation are genuine. The client's 'story' attempts to explain the experience. For example, the practitioner could reply 'you must be very frightened by this'. The practitioner has not agreed with the client's story but has empathized and reflected back possible feelings about it: 'it must be very depressing for you'; 'do you get lonely here?'. These responses are likely to produce a reduction in the expression of the delusional belief and increase discussion of the actual situation and feelings about it as meetings progress.

At times the expression of delusions may be too acute or too well established. It may not always be possible to build a rapport with the client in these situations until appropriate medication has been administered. ✱Psychotrophic medication controls rather than 'cures' delusions. With medication the client's delusions are less likely to be overtly expressed even though they may still lie just beneath the surface. The practitioner may have more success in communicating when the client's anxieties are eased by medication.

When treating psychotic delusions a dual approach to care would seem appropriate, with both medical intervention and supportive therapy. The practitioner will be well placed to observe and monitor the effects of medication.

DEPRESSION (see also Delusions; Behavioural psychotherapy)

A depressed mood can be a secondary component of other psychiatric disorders or physical illnesses. When it is the primary disorder the traditional medical model divides the condition into two clinical categories:

1. reactive (neurotic) depression
2. endogenous (psychotic) depression.

Reactive depression, as the term suggests, is seen as an exaggerated reaction to an external stressor. That is to say, there is always a precipitating event (such as the loss of a loved one) or environmental factors which are instrumental in the development of the illness' (Brooking et al., 1992).

Endogenous depression may arise out of the blue, is characterized by more severe depression, without reactivity, with guilt, and pessimism which may reach delusional intensity. There is also a view that depression is a continuum with reactive at one pole and endogenous at the other' (Fottrell, 1983).

The practitioner may see an overlap of symptoms between these types of depression particularly when working with the elderly. The 'continuum model' may span grief reactions, agitated/paranoid presentations and pseudo-dementia. When carrying out an assessment of a depressive disorder the practitioner may find it helpful to consider using the following steps (Gelder et al., 1994).

1. Verify diagnosis
2. Assess severity
3. Assess causes
4. Assess social resources
5. Assess effects on others.

Verify diagnosis

The practitioner is able to aid the diagnostic process by thorough history-taking that includes the client's view of the problem. Many clients emphasize the physical symptoms of their depression, including poor appetite or sleep, lack of energy, weight loss or gastrointestinal complaints and this can 'mask' the depressive illness. Conversely, a depression may be secondary to organic causes, including infections, endocrine disorders, carcinoma and the dementias. Drugs can also cause depression, particularly the antihypotensives, corticosteroids, anticonvulsants, oral contraceptives and some neuroleptics. In 'neurotic' depression, anxiety is often a feature. Clients may be so neglected in appearance or retarded in speech or movement. They are usually more able to give a full account of their history and problems. Clients often have difficulty in getting off to sleep and their mood is usually lower in the evening. Poor appetite and weight loss are not so commonly seen in this milder form of depression. The expression of delusions or hallucinations would indicate the more severe diagnosis of 'psychotic' depression. The content of the client's statements about themselves is usually negative and involves feelings and ideas of guilt, worthlessness, perceived ill health or poverty and persecution. Speech is often slow or monosyllabic. Self-neglect and psychomotor agitation or retardation can be observed. The mood tends to be lower first thing in the morning with a slight improvement as the day goes on. Unlike the neurotic depressive disorders where clients will tell the practitioner about how unhappy or anxious they feel, in severe depressive disorders clients may say that they feel no emotion. These assessment findings will prove invaluable for the diagnostic and treatment options.

Assess severity

The severity of the depression is assessed by both the practitioner's observations and the reports of the carers. Delusions and hallucinations, vastly reduced involvement in work, family and social activities and the expression of suicidal thoughts are all indications of a more severe form of depression. It is important to remember that suicide may occur during recovery from a depressive disorder in clients who, when more severely depressed, had thought of the act but lacked the initiative to carry it out (Gelder et al., 1994). Other suicide risk factors to be aware of are alcohol or drug dependence, isolation, chronic pain and older age.

Assess causes

The assessment of causes will enable the practitioner to plan intervention. Concerns about physical health will need to be passed on to the client's doctor. When implementing treatment, the practitioner may have to work using more than one approach or model. A biomedical model will involve the practitioner in monitoring the effects of medication, encouraging compliance and observing and reporting on the client's mental state. In parallel to this, the practitioner may use treatment approaches derived from psychological or sociological models. Examples of these interventions are as follows.

- **Cognitive–behavioural therapy** – the practitioner challenges the validity of the client's thoughts by applying reason and logic. This is a problem-solving approach that complements the nursing process framework.
- **Psychosocial counselling** – exploration of coping skills and life events are the focus for discussion.
- **Counselling** – these approaches can range from simple advice-giving, to the client-centred or psychodynamic. However, in general therapeutic counselling is based on the development of an understanding relationship within which clients can help themselves to change (Brooking *et al.*, 1992).

Assess social resources

While family, friends, or work may have a very important role in the client's recovery and support network, it must be recognized that they may also be a source of stress for the client. The practitioner will need to liaise closely to advise, educate and support carers.

Assess effects on others

The practitioner should be aware of the potential for neglect or harm to others when a client is severely depressed. Delusional thoughts may lead the client to carry out 'mercy killings' on their children to prevent them 'suffering also', or for a client to kill their spouse due to pathological jealousy. The practitioner will be aware of the role of the psychiatric day hospital and the psychiatric outpatient clinic as extra resources for the monitoring and treatment of their client's depression. When the client's depression is not responding to treatment, there is severe self-neglect, or a high risk of suicide or homicide, then inpatient treatment on a psychiatric ward will need to be arranged by the psychiatrist. Electro-convulsive treatment may need to be given while a client is an inpatient, but for some years this treatment has also been available for outpatient status.

DIFFUSING ANGER

There are two aspects to this. Firstly, the practitioner needs to find strategies that will help in directly diffusing the anger that may be presented by the client, and secondly, to help the client to discover schemes that can be employed in controlling anger in daily life. The use of verbal techniques that help to diffuse anger is very effective. By observation, the practitioner can assess the way in which anger is building up in the client. For example, the client may display facial expressions or body movements that suggest strong feelings and the practitioner can then directly intervene verbally. For example, it is helpful to acknowledge the client's feelings in ways such as 'I can see that you are feeling angry right now. Can we stop and talk about it?'. Reflecting on what has been talked about prior to the appearance of angry feelings is also useful in clarifying what is happening. The practitioner could reflect aloud 'it seems that something we have been talking about has made you feel very uncomfortable. Could you tell me a bit more about what it is that has upset you?' This also gives the practitioner the opportunity to check what is happening in the relationship and to reflect on his or her own behaviour towards the client which may contribute towards the growth of angry feelings. For example, the practitioner may have made some false assumptions which the client interprets as judgemental or patronizing and these need to be corrected. When the anger has been diffused the practitioner can also check with the client whether there are any other factors that are causing concern that may need to be explored before the practitioner closes the session.

DISCHARGE FROM HOSPITAL (*see also* Admission; Advocacy; Labelling; Care Programme Approach, Supervision registers)

When planning the discharge of a client from a psychiatric hospital, the ward team will consider the transfer of the individual care plan from hospital to the community. To ensure continuity of care, provision has to be made for follow-up support, monitoring and therapy. The choices open to the ward team are:

- discharge back to the care of the general practitioner;
- attendance at a psychiatric day hospital or outpatient clinic;
- the allocation of a mental health practitioner/keyworker such as a community psychiatric nurse.

Follow-up care may involve any combination of the above choices. If a community practitioner was not involved prior to the admission, one will probably be allocated during a ward meeting. A successful package of care will be facilitated by the practitioner liaising in the first instance with the client's keyworker on the ward and by attending ward meetings. Prior to discharge, the practitioner will also need to liaise and work jointly with colleagues from other disciplines who have input into pre-discharge and follow-up plans. By meeting the client's relatives and other informal carers, previous care involvement can be reinstated and enhanced.

The longer clients are in hospital the more difficult it can be for them to reintegrate into family and social roles. There may be loss of status when previous roles are taken over by others and there is reluctance to hand these back to the 'patient' during perceived 'convalescence'. A combination of the individual's loss of confidence and negative attitudes by others towards mental illness may make it harder to re-engage socially.

Community mental health practitioners have an important role in supporting clients and their families and facilitating positive communications between them. They also have an advocate role whereby they assist in mobilizing community resources on behalf of their clients. When the practitioner is a community psychiatric nurse, an additional role will be the monitoring and administration of medications and observation of the individual's mental health. If the client is to be cared for under the provision of the care programme or supervision register procedures then the practitioner may have the added responsibility of ensuring these are implemented and that regular review meetings are arranged.

DISORIENTATION (*see also* Delusions; Hallucinations; Reality orientation)

When we are orientated, we are aware of the time and date, where we are, who we are, and who our relatives and friends are. It is normal to be temporarily disorientated when we are in unfamiliar environments but our judgement and reasoning enables us to re-orientate ourselves. In situations where stimuli and cues are reduced, such as darkness, social isolation or sensory deprivation, disorientation can be increased. Orientation is a function of the sense organs and the perceptual processes which accompany them. In organic brain syndromes these processes are disordered and the sufferer may experience a distorted sense of time and be unable to orientate himself in terms of place. He may be unable to say who he is or to recognize relatives or significant others (Sugden *et al.*, 1986). One of the clinical features of Alzheimer's disease is progressive disorientation where early signs can be evident when the person is in unfamiliar surroundings, for example on holiday (Gelder *et al.*, 1994). Due to impairment of perception, memory and reasoning, the person finds it increasingly difficult to re-orientate by using the cues in the environment. The person may be driving a car and for the first time not recognize the local roads leading to home. The driving skills remain but the 'mental map' is lost and the passenger, by necessity, becomes the 'navigator'. Disorientation for time and, at a later stage, for place and person are almost invariable once dementia is well established (Gelder *et al.*, 1994). Disorientation for time may be the cause of nocturnal wandering, reverse sleep pattern, wanting to go out at night or refusing to go to bed. Later, disorientation for place may occur, when failure to recognize their own home results in the sufferer asking the carer 'when are we going home?'

They may not be able to find the toilet or their bedroom even though they may have lived in the same house for many years. In residential homes it is common for sufferers to go into other residents' rooms while searching for familiar cues. Disorientation of person may bring about the situation whereby the sufferer does not even recognize their partner and perceives them to be a stranger, a nurse or even a parent. A degree of disorientation can also occur in the acute organic states including hypoglycaemia, dehydration and other metabolic disorders. Added physical problems will exacerbate disorientation in a person already suffering a chronic organic disorder. Practitioners can take an educative approach when working in partnership with carers. By explaining the nature of disorientation, carers will gain more understanding of the client's experiences and perhaps carer tolerance levels will increase. Together, practitioners and carers can explore the causes of disorientation and seek ways of reducing its impact. By controlling the environment, carers may be able to increase cues and stimuli and reduce the risk of accident. When clients are restless and wandering, falls are more likely to occur and there is always the possibility of clients wandering out of their homes. In the client's own home the environment may be more familiar but disorientation can still occur, especially at night when light is poor. 'Reality orientation' (RO) techniques can be taught to carers and usefully applied in the client's own home. RO is intended to maintain reality contact and to reverse or halt confusion, disorientation, social withdrawal and apathy (Brooking *et al.*, 1992). Orientation cues are provided, for instance clocks, calendars, photographs and names of rooms on doors. Regular discussions on topical issues in newspapers and repeated updating on family matters will help to keep clients in touch with reality. While under-stimulation may not provide enough cues, over-stimulation can provide too many ambiguous cues. Television or radio may provide a focus for discussion, but neither are helpful in the background when other discussion is taking place. Where possible, clients should be included in conversation rather than being left to keep up with it. It can be very wearing for carers when clients keep asking the same questions and answers have to be repeated. Saying 'I have already told you where you are' is not going to help as tensions will rise. Repetition and extreme patience are needed to maintain the client's orientation and carers will require much moral support and advice from practitioners.

DOCUMENTATION

One of the most common reasons for nurses finding themselves facing disciplinary hearings at the Professional Conduct Committee of the UKCC is inaccurate or inadequate clinical record keeping. In 1991, 31 nurses were struck off the register for poor record keeping; a significant proportion of nurses finding themselves in this position work in the community.

The importance of accurate, timely and relevant clinical records cannot be overstated. However, with monotonous regularity, public enquiries, reports from health service ombudsman and clinical audit reports describe serious problems in the quality of clinical records. The chief nurse at the NHS Executive, Mrs Yvonne Moores, in the cover note of *Keeping the Records Straight, A Guide to Record Keeping for Nurses, Midwives and Health Visitors* published in 1993 by the NHS Training Directorate states:

> The fundamental importance of record keeping as a foundation of care cannot be emphasized too strongly. Accurate, complete and up to date records represent a vital component of high quality care. Some of the messages and real life examples outlined in the course are deliberately shocking particularly when the potential consequences of poor records are examined. It is therefore important not to lose sight of the other side of the coin – the tangible and positive benefits that high quality records bring – to patients, clients and their relatives, to nurses, midwives and health visitors and to the health service as a whole.

This document considers legal issues, professional discipline, workload issues, care and quality issues and examples of records by specialism including community nursing and mental health nursing. The examples given contain some of the most common problems found in clinical records. These include:

- sections being left blank rather than marked as not applicable;
- illegible entries;
- entries not signed or dated;
- entries being initialled rather than signed;
- signatures being illegible;
- signatures not including the designation of the nurse;
- entries made by untrained or learner nurses not being countersigned by a trained nurse;
- the use of abbreviations or jargon;
- errors being erased with Tipp-ex;
- inconsistencies between the assessed problem and the planned intervention;
- problems being described in a care plan without an associated intervention;
- lack of review dates on care plans.

The Health Service Commissioner's annual report 1992/93 is quoted in *Just for the Record A Guide for Record Keeping for Health Care Professionals* published by the NHS Training Directorate in 1994. An extract states:

Careful attention to record keeping is not just a matter of good practice, it is integral to the provision and continuity of good care. But at its lowest, it is an insurance for a member of staff who may later be accused of negligence. What do I find? In too many cases records are incomplete or lacking in essential detail. In others there is no record of communication with relatives or carers, or of discharge arrangements. Even if records are well maintained they are of no use if they cannot be found when they are needed.

This quotation introduces the additional concept of care of clinical records and again all too often records are 'lost'.

One of the most common problems found when community mental health nurses' clinical records are audited is that the records have not been maintained contemporaneously. Many community mental health nurses still see record keeping as an administrative burden which consumes valuable time which could be better spent delivering care to clients. In April 1993 the UKCC published *Standards for Records and Record Keeping*. The introduction to this pamphlet states:

The important activity of making and keeping records is an essential and integral part of care and not a distraction from its provision. There is, however, substantial evidence to indicate that inadequate and inappropriate record keeping concerning the care of patients and clients neglects their interest through:

1.1   impairing continuity of care;
1.2   introducing discontinuity of communication between staff;
1.3   creating the risk of medication or other treatments being duplicated or omitted.
1.4   failing to focus attention on early signs of deviation from the norm;
1.5   failing to place on record significant alterations and conclusions.

Both *Keeping the Record Straight* and *Just for the Record* provide a template for good practice and record keeping. They suggest that clinical records should be:

- understandable
- accurate
- complete
- consistent
- up to date
- relevant
- coherent
- clear

- timely/contemporaneous
- legible
- personalized
- respectful of the patients/clients
- concise.

The rationale for each of these elements should be self-evident; however, more detailed explanations for each are contained in *Standards for Records and Record Keeping* issued by the UKCC. Copies of this document can be obtained free from the UKCC and all community mental health nurses would be well advised to obtain a copy if they do not already have one. Arguably the most important part of this document is the summary of principles underpinning records and these are as follows.

41   The following principles must apply.
41.1 The record is directed primarily in serving the interest of the patient or client to whom it relates and enabling the provision of care, the prevention of disease and the promotion of health.
41.2 The record demonstrates the accurate chronology of events and all significant consultations, assessments, observations, decisions, interventions and outcomes.
41.3 The record and the activity of record keeping is an integral and essential part of care and not a distraction from its provision.
41.4 The record is clear and unambiguous.
41.5 The record contains entries recording facts and observations written at the time of, or soon after, the events described.
41.6 The record provides a safe and effective means of communication between members of the health care team and supports continuity of care.
41.7 The record demonstrates that the practitioner's duty of care has been fulfilled.
41.8 The systems for record keeping exclude unauthorized access of breaches of confidentiality.
41.9 The record is constructed and completed in such a manner as to facilitate the monitoring of standards, audit, quality assurance and the investigation of complaints.

The principles outlined above should guide all clinical record keeping by community mental health nurses. We must ensure that nursing records accurately reflect the quality and detail of the clinical care being provided. *Keeping the Record Straight* contains a case study from 1992 describing how a district nurse with 17 years' experience was struck off with immediate effect for failing to record assessments and care plan details about a particular client. In *Just for the Record* there is a quotation from a health visitor:

As a health visitor with a heavy case load I just felt I had too much to do, but I couldn't convince my supervisor of it. For a year I kept a record of everything I couldn't do but I should be doing. Shortly after they appointed a part time health visitor to take part of my case load.

The answer to record keeping problems is in practitioners' own hands.

DRAMA TECHNIQUES (*see also* Bereavement; Communication and Relationship-building techniques)

The use of drama techniques is a powerful aid to expressing feelings which the client may find difficult to articulate. The verbalization of deep seated feelings is often difficult for the client. They may feel ashamed of expressing anger, for example, or may be afraid that what they say will shock or embarrass the practitioner. For many people, their expression of feeling is influenced by how they were encouraged to show emotions while growing up, reinforced by peer groups, the media and other factors. The use of drama techniques is often a powerful aid to expressing these feelings. However, it is important that the client and practitioner are already working together in a warm supportive relationship where the client will view the practitioner with trust; obviously the practitioner will have knowledge of whether this type of work will benefit the client and whether the idea will not cause dismay. The type of clients for whom this may not be beneficial are the acutely psychotic and those whose view of themselves is diffuse. However, those for whom it may be of great benefit are those who have suffered a loss and who are able to articulate this.

Specific techniques that can be used are as follows. Firstly, the client who has suffered and is finding it hard to express feelings about that loss can be encouraged to imagine that the object of loss is sitting in a chair opposite them, and be asked to talk to that object. This often produces very strong results once the client has become used to the idea, and often the predominant feeling expressed is anger. Secondly, the same process can be used with the client using a cushion to hold and talk to. This may be particularly appropriate for the client who has lost a child, as the action of holding will release memories that may not have surfaced. Thirdly, role play can also be used on a one to one basis, or with a group, perhaps to practise assertive techniques or to look at one's behaviour in relation to someone else. Feedback from the client about the whole experience will be helpful for the practitioner, to evaluate the possibility of future work.

E

ELDERLY MENTAL HEALTH SERVICES (*see also* Working base; Carers)

Our elderly population has been steadily increasing since the start of this century, and the UK has one of the oldest populations in the world. Between 1971 and 1981 the number of people of pensionable age rose by a million and it is predicted that from now to the end of this century there will be an increase in the proportion of elderly who survive past the age of 85 years (Central Statistical Office, 1984). Community mental health practitioners working generically are likely to have a significant proportion of elderly on their caseloads. Some mental health teams are now specializing in the areas of drug and alcohol abuse, rehabilitation, children, family therapy, crisis work or the elderly. The two CPNA surveys of 1980 and 1985 found that the largest area of specialist work of CPNs is with the elderly, with one in five CPNs working with this client group (Community Psychiatric Nurses Association, 1980, 1985). With estimates for the incidence of dementia being 10% for those over 65 and 20% for those over 80 years (Health Advisory Service, 1982), one can see why the mental health services are giving priority to this specialization. Mental health teams specializing in the mental health of the elderly are varied in their structure, referral criteria and working bases. Some teams only accept referrals for clients with an organic illness while other teams also accept those with a functional illness. Teams can differ in their age criteria for accepting referrals, for instance only accepting referrals for those over the age of 75 years. The elderly are often described as having 'multifactorial problems' that may be physical, mental, social or financial. Under these headings the individual may experience sensory impairment, poor mobility, bereavement, social deprivation and loss of independence. Ideally, a mental health team for the elderly will be multidisciplinary, where joint assessments and co-working facilitates a more holistic approach to meeting the needs of their elderly clients. In many areas, the social services employ care managers who work specifically with the elderly to provide practical and personal care and support (care packages) that enable the elderly person to live as independently as possible in their own home. Community mental health practitioners are able to complement this care package by providing mental health assessment and advice for the care managers on mental health issues including symptoms, mood, behaviour and medication. In addition to the community mental health team, the services for the elderly mentally ill include outpatient clinics, psychiatric day hospitals, assessment wards in the hospitals and high dependency units. The social services provide day centres, respite beds and permanent residential care for the elderly. In some areas this care is 'enhanced' to cater for the elderly with mental health problems. In the private sector there are residential/nursing homes that are registered to cater for the needs of the elderly mentally ill; in some cases these are providing day and respite care. When working with clients with a functional diagnosis, practitioners may work in a similar way to their generic colleagues. The elderly experience the same range of mental health problems as younger people and likewise will require help for anxiety, depression, phobias, obsessions, schizophrenia or mania. Clients suffering organic mental health problems such as dementia require a different approach and service. The practitioner tends to work more in partnership with the carer to enable them to continue caring, but with support and advice.

EMOTIONAL EFFECTS OF PHYSICAL ILLNESS (*see also* Side effects of medication)

Although there is increasing focus on the effects of stress and anxiety on body systems, recognition needs also to be made of the effects of physical illness on the emotions. The holistic approach to nursing means that it is equally as important to assess the physical and psychological elements of illness. Rowden (1993) makes the point that for example, a confirmed diagnosis of terminal illness given to someone who already has emotional problems with which they are coping, is seen as 'the last straw' and may cause a crisis of severe anxiety or depression. The same may be true for the client with severe pain related to chronic illness such as arthritis. Elderly clients particularly may suffer depression caused by increasing difficulties with mobility which increases their isolation and frustration. Physical treatments may also cause emotional distress which is not always admitted to by the client or easily recognized by the professional; the value of careful assessment of the total person is therefore of importance.

EMPOWERMENT

The term empowerment has been driven into mental health care from active service user groups, to confront the effects of institutionalization on those persons experiencing mental health difficulties. Institutionalization can be seen as affecting both practitioners and clients and the drive for health professionals to empower clients is reflected both through practitioners' governing bodies push to encourage practitioners to empower themselves and take more responsibility for their care (UKCC, 1984a; 1984b) and through a Government drive to encourage all persons to take responsibility for their health (Patients' Charter, 1995). This may be a positive move but in order for empowerment of the individual to occur, certain criteria must be met:

- practitioners should feel empowered themselves – able to act with authority and autonomy;
- practitioners should ensure that their clients feel able to cope with being empowered;
- practitioners *cannot* empower others but can facilitate others to empower themselves. It is not a basket of surprises to be passed around but a way of feeling and believing;
- clients need to understand what empowerment entails and to take their own time in gaining the skills to enable their own empowerment.

Example

A client's medication should be discussed fully at each meeting. The client should be made aware through educative processes of such issues as the side effects, dosage, long-term prospects and opportunities to reduce their dosage. This can be done by fully involving the client and giving all the information about their medication, allowing them the opportunity to make an *informed choice* about their chemical treatment. Enabling the client to make informed choices is an excellent demonstration of the way a practitioner can enable the client to become empowered and make decisions about their life and treatment.

EVALUATION

The nature of community mental health work results in the development of close relationships with clients and this helps in the work of evaluating the care that is being given and the progress that the client is making. Each practitioner needs to identify the method of evaluation that will be used, that is when it will take place, to what extent self-evaluation by the client can be used and how it will be recorded by all those involved in the process. The client can be encouraged, for example, to keep a diary or to use daily rating scales that demonstrate fluctuations in mood or activity; these will then be of great use in identifying the extent to which outcomes are being met. Summarizing and analysing the data received from all available sources (client, family and others involved in care) will result in the setting of new or modified objectives in the nursing care plan. Continual evaluation also enables the practitioner to check that the goals set with and for the client, whether short or long term, are realistic, since this will be evident during evaluation. Again, working closely with the client in this process enables both client and practitioner to take pride in the successes achieved and to work together on the areas that are causing problems.

FAMILY THERAPY

Family therapy utilizes the family concepts found in role, developmental and systems theories. It provides intervention when family interaction patterns have become too rigid and helps the family to find solutions. Family therapy interventions have in common:

- the assessment of the family system as a whole;
- the focus on the process of the family's interactions;
- the shaping of goals;
- the confronting of dysfunctional patterns (Hershenson and Power, 1987).

However, within this common framework, therapists may have different approaches to helping families such as the 'psychodynamic' approach of Akerman (1966), the 'communication' approach of Haley (1976), or the 'structural' approach of Minuchin (1974). In some areas family therapists operate as a multidisciplinary team and conduct the therapy within a purpose-built suite. One or two members of the team take on the role of interviewers and facilitate the session while colleagues observe through a one-way screen. The session is usually recorded on video to enable the team to study the session between family appointments. A telephone links the observers with the interviewers to enable spontaneous interventions to be made or to call colleagues back for supervision. White boards are often used in either or both rooms to construct family genograms or to write down intervention ideas or important issues raised. Family therapists prefer to observe and understand the context in which a behaviour exists rather than the context of the behaviour itself. They find it useful to study a sequence of behaviour and not focus on a single piece of behaviour, thereby shifting emphasis from 'symptom-bearer' (or patient) to a broader picture. Knowledge of what constitutes a healthy family system is useful as it enables the team to centre on unhealthy issues such as:

• unclear communication, perception, boundaries or responsibilities;
• rigid adherence to redundant solutions;
• alienated or enmeshed family members.

It is often within these areas that many mental health problems exist. Family therapy shifts the emphasis from symptom/diagnostic label to problem/behaviour, for instance 'I am an agoraphobic' to 'I experience anxiety when out alone'. The use of the 'W' questions helps the family to see problems rather than illness.

• 'Who is the problem?'
• 'Why is that a problem?'
• 'Who is it a problem for?'
• 'When is it a problem?
• 'Where is it a problem?'
• 'What have you tried to do about it?'

Family therapy aims to encourage healthy open communication and identify what needs to change. Many of the problem exploration and intervention techniques used by family therapists can be useful in mental health counselling and study of family therapy theories will help the practitioner gain a wider understanding of clients' problems and family dynamics.

G

GETTING IN (INITIAL VISIT) (*see also* Appointments)

If the appointments procedure has been followed then the client should already have some expectation as to the reason for the visit. An initial visit introduction may well proceed as follows.

1. A check by the practitioner that they have the correct client and address.
2. The practitioner displaying their identity card.
3. The practitioner giving their name and title.
4. The practitioner enquiring as to whether the client received the appointment and was expecting the visit.
5. If necessary a brief reminder of the reason for the visit, for instance 'your doctor asked me to visit you'.

Usually the practitioner is invited in well before stage 5 is reached.

In an outpatient clinic situation, the client travels to the practitioner and the interview takes place in the practitioner's territory. There is usually a mutual, albeit unspoken, expectation: 'I have come here to see if you can help me'; 'You have come to see me so I assume you are motivated to seek my help'.

The initial rapport is formalized in the clinic setting and the practitioner retains control. In the home visiting situation, the boot is on the other foot: 'I have come to offer help'; 'I don't know yet if I want your help'. We are now in the client's territory.

If practitioners have been sent rather than asked for, if clients are suspicious, withdrawn, confused, over-anxious or are suffering from delusions, paranoid ideas or mania, then practitioners could well find that they are not immediately invited in.

In the main, the offer of help is welcome and getting out can be more of a problem than getting in.

When first contact, on the doorstep, indicates that this may be the shortest home visit ever, then now is the moment when the practitioner's skills are most tested. One minute is a very short time in which to reassure the anxious, motivate the withdrawn, orientate the confused, calm the euphoric or convince the psychotic that they are here to help.

'You seem concerned by the referral, perhaps using this opportunity to talk might help?'

This statement conveys empathy. The practitioner is seen to recognize the client's apprehension and accepts the validity of it. The offer of help is put forward tentatively rather than authoritatively. Clients may decide that this 'opportunity' is a chance to air their own views and to check what practitioners have to offer and whether they can be trusted.

The skills of remaining overtly unshaken (even if covertly stirred), of conveying acceptance and maintaining the offer of help in acute situations usually succeed in showing the client that this practitioner is not easily diverted from their objective.

This display of self assurance and experience can create, for the client, an initial feeling of confidence in the practitioner, and at least a willingness to consider help. The start of a relationship as expressed in words: 'you might as well come in then'.

GOAL SETTING

Goal setting is possibly the most vital stage of the nursing process, relying on thorough assessment and the ability of the client and practitioner to work closely together in a supportive relationship. The information gained during the assessment interviews will indicate the direction in which the client can move in the achievement of a desirable goal, and this can be used not just by the client and practitioner but also by others who appear relevantly involved in the life of the client. There are several important issues to consider when formulating goals or objectives. Nelson-Jones (1988) points out that decisions about goals inevitably involve values, not just those of the client but, more importantly, of the practitioner. They may not have the same values or points of view regarding future movements, but they do need to be compatible to avoid producing objectives that are incompatible with the feelings and beliefs of the client. Secondly, any objective must be attainable and written in such a way that the client can identify a time span for its success. For example, to write 'John will feel less tense' is not particularly helpful nor positive sounding, nor can John see how he can achieve what may be a highly desirable outcome. To write, however, 'John will do half an hour of relaxation exercises after work' gives John an outcome which is measurable, can be achieved and which he understands will contribute to the overcoming of his tension. Statements used in the writing should always be measurable and also, most importantly, they should be positive so that the client can see what he or she can achieve, and not just what will diminish. It is, therefore, far more encouraging to read 'Ann will go to the day centre on Mondays' than to read 'Ann will not stay indoors watching television in the day time'. As Ward (1985, page 60) states: 'Positive statements imply that the patient is learning to use more effective personal strategies, whilst negative ones imply that he is simply not to use old and ineffective ones. One offers alternatives, the other highlights failure'. It is also important to note the difference between internal and external goals and to ensure that both are considered and planned for. Internal goals are those which the client states as his own, often in terms of a problem in need of resolution such as 'I don't know anyone on this estate and I feel as though I'll go mad if I spend any more time on my own'. External goals are those provided for the client by others and the two types should be compatible in providing a full and achievable future plan. Finally, it is important that the language used is that of the client, avoiding jargon or technical terms that may merely be confusing.

Objectives may be written as behavioural or expressive statements, depending on the needs of the client. Behavioural objectives are used where achievement in some type of action needs to be demonstrated and where the client will be able to see time-specific, quantifiable statements that he or she can see being achieved. So 'Ann will get the bus to the day centre on Mondays' tells Ann exactly what will be happening and how. Expressive objectives, on the other hand, look at the thought processes that are going on behind the behaviour and therefore they are often used together. The client, as well as being encouraged to achieve the desired changes in behaviour, is also given the opportunity to look at the more emotional/psychological side of the behaviours with statements such as 'John will keep a daily diary for the next week to describe how he feels before and after he has done the relaxation exercises and this will be discussed with Jane next week'.

Each problem area identified should therefore have an objective linked to it, as realistic and specific as possible, so that it is obvious at a glance what the client has to do and what can be achieved by so doing. Once goals have been identified, the practitioner and client can work together to prioritize them, and also to identify which are short-term and which are long-term goals. It is important when prioritizing, that factors such as culture or environment are taken into account, since these may influence the successful achievement of the goals. For the client to 'own' his or her set of objectives, it is obvious that they need to be formulated with as much input from the client and relevant others as possible and regular discussion should take place to ensure that, at all times, they meet the client's needs and demonstrate to him or her a view of the positive change that can take place.

H

HALLUCINATIONS (*see also* Delusions, Disorientation)

'A hallucination is a perception experienced in the absence of an external stimulus to the corresponding sense organ, for example, hearing a voice when no one is speaking within hearing distance' (Gelder *et al.*, 1994). Hallucinations can be part of the normal experience particularly just prior to falling asleep or when waking, but these tend to be brief and orientation soon follows. Hallucinations can occur in any of the sensory modes with auditory (hearing) and visual hallucinations being the most common. Olfactory (smell), gustatory (taste) and tactile (touch) hallucinations, though less common, do present in some mental disorders. A person experiencing auditory hallucinations may hear noises, music or voices. Examples of visual hallucinations are flashes of light, animals or people. The smells and tastes of the olfactory and gustatory hallucinations are most often experienced as unpleasant. Complaints of insects crawling under the skin or of being touched or sexually interfered with are sometimes expressed by the person suffering tactile hallucinations.

Hallucinations, usually visual, can be present in the acute organic states where perception is affected by various underlying causes including alcohol, drugs, infections, carcinoma or head injury. Less marked perceptual disorders (illusions) may occur in the organic disorders. 'Illusions are misinterpretations of external stimuli. They occur when sensory input is restricted, for example in poor light or low levels of audibility' (Gelder *et al.*, 1994). Visual hallucinations are less common than auditory hallucinations in the functional psychoses of schizophrenia and manic depression. In schizophrenia, the sufferer experiences a disorder of perception where auditory hallucinations are characteristic of the diagnosis. Hallucinatory voices may take the form of a running commentary on an individual's behaviour, or the voices may give instructions. In some cases, two or more voices may talk about the sufferer in the third person. The less common tactile, olfactory and gustatory hallucinations occur mainly in schizophrenia. In severe depressive disorders, voices may be heard as repetitive words or phrases with the content supporting the individual's delusional ideas of unworthiness or guilt. Olfactory hallucinations may occur in some people who become severely depressed, with the individual being convinced that they emit an odour. In mania, hallucinations are usually consistent with the mood, taking the form of a voice speaking to the client about his special powers or, occasionally, visions with a religious content (Gelder *et al.*, 1994).

The terms hallucination, delusion, illusion and disorientation can sometimes be incorrectly applied to the client's behaviour. When accurately applied, these observations can assist the diagnostic process and choice of treatment options. In the acute organic states, knowledge of physical causes will enable the practitioner to take on a preventative and advisory role. The elderly in particular are prone to acute toxic confusion caused by drugs, infections and even constipation. In the chronic organic states (dementia) where toxins can exacerbate an already confused state, the practitioner may work closely with the carer in monitoring medications and providing advice on health issues such as diet and fluid intake. Hallucinations and illusions can occur in the chronic organic states and it is helpful for the practitioner to explain to the client and carer what is happening and to explore ways of responding to these events. The practitioner can find out if the client is distressed by the hallucinations, for instance 'strange men in the bedroom', or just mildly interested; 'the child sitting in the chair opposite'.

Is the carer getting unnecessarily upset and trying too hard to convince the client that, for instance, the child is not really there? If the client is not unduly worried then diversional tactics such as changing the subject or introducing an activity may help. If the client is distressed then getting them to shout at the hallucination to 'go away', or to turn their back to it, can sometimes be effective. If the problem is very distressing and persistent then medication may be prescribed to calm the agitation associated with the hallucination. It could be helpful to consider lighting in the home if the client has poor eyesight as hallucinations may be the result of misinterpretation and/or disorientation. Carers can often be frightened themselves when clients describe hallucinations and their anxiety can be 'infectious'. By explaining the nature of these experiences, the practitioner may enable the carer to use a reassuring approach to the client when these events occur. In the functional psychoses, the client can be deeply convinced by their experiences and not so easily reassured or diverted. Tactful enquiry should be made as to whether the client is experiencing hallucinations. The subject can be introduced by the practitioner saying 'when the nerves are upset some people have unusual experiences'. Questions can then be asked about hearing voices or seeing unusual things (Gelder *et al.*, 1994). By empathizing with the client's concerns, attempting to explain and reassure and exploring techniques for coping, the therapeutic relationship can be enhanced. Trust and confidence in the practitioner will be built on acceptance rather than argument as to whether the client's perceptions are real or not: the client's anxieties will be real enough. The practitioner should look for any evidence of trigger factors that might predispose towards hallucinations, for example when, where or with whom do these events take place? The practitioner should monitor medication and confirm this is being taken correctly. Medication needs to be reviewed if distressing symptoms do not seem to be alleviated.

HEALTH OF THE NATION

The Department of Health (1994) identified five key areas in its White Paper *The Health of the Nation*. These five key areas included:

- HIV and AIDS
- mental illness
- coronary heart disease and stroke
- cancers
- accidents.

This section will offer an overview of the key area of mental illness.

Three targets were set in the 1994 publication, two relating to the reduction of suicide rates and the third to improving the health and social functioning of mentally ill people. According to the publication *The Health of the Nation, One Year On* (DoH, 1995), the suicide rate increased slightly for 1990–1992 and the objective of suicide reduction continues to be an objective for the year 2000. Additionally areas for targeting include the implementation of the Care Programme Approach, supervision register, primary care, the development of comprehensive local services and the development of prevention strategies in the workplace.

The Health of the Nation (DoH, 1994a) and the *Mental Illness Key Area Handbook* (DoH, 1994c) outline information on how local services could act together to achieve the targets and offer a reflection on the profile of mental health. Both are useful reading to understand the rationale for workplace managerial and Government initiatives.

HIV POSITIVE AND HEPATITIS B – ADMINISTRATION OF MEDICINE (*see also* HIV/AIDS and mental health)

It is the responsibility of practitioners to update themselves with regard to current practice on a number of issues; none more so than in the case of human immune deficiency virus and hepatitis B antigen patients. As both these viruses are present in blood and other bodily fluids, it is necessary when administering medication parenterally (either intermuscularly or intravenously) for precautions to be taken. It is important that all practitioners be up to date with current guidelines for managing contact with people who are HIV/hepatitis B positive and people thought to be HIV/hepatitis B positive (DHSS, 1986; USDSS, 1988).

The Standards for the Administration of Medicines (UKCC, 1992) must be followed at all times. With a client who is HIV positive, gloves should be worn when administering medicine via injection and if the client should bleed on withdrawal of the needle, the practitioner should apply direct pressure with a sterile swab. The needle and syringe should be disposed of in a separate bin labelled 'High Risk' for waste from HIV positive or hepatitis B antigen positive patients. For further information on administering medicine see Ritter (1989).

HIV/AIDS AND MENTAL HEALTH

In 1989, the Royal College of Psychiatrists identified that clients with a diagnosis of HIV/AIDS would increasingly require community mental health care. The main groups who require mental health care are those with:

• primarily a mental health diagnosis and an HIV diagnosis;
• HIV diagnosis and mental health needs directly related to this;
• AIDS-related brain impairment.

Clients who have primary diagnosis of a severe mental illness who then become HIV positive will require much support from the community mental health practitioner. The practitioner should have a knowledge and awareness of the potential effects of an HIV diagnosis, along with an understanding of the development of the illness. The client's mental health needs should be met as usual but the practitioner needs to consider the effects of the HIV diagnosis and allow time for the client to talk about it, with the practitioner checking their understanding. The practitioner should ensure that expert advice and support can be accessed as and when required for both themselves and the client. All protective measures should be taken as stated in local and national policy when dealing with any bodily fluids of the client.

Clients who are diagnosed as HIV positive who have little or no contact with the mental health services may develop mental health needs in relation to their diagnosis. Many individuals suffer from adjustment reactions, but these may be limited in time. Long-term responses such as depression are less common. Psychosocial reactions to potentially fatal conditions are similar but in the case of HIV and AIDS are magnified by the stigma attached to it and by the fears of social rejection. Psychiatric disturbance is greatest immediately after diagnosis and in the later stages of the disease.

The Royal College of Psychiatrists (1989) suggests that major depression and adjustment reactions are the main disorders.

In many clients AIDS-related brain impairment has been described; this chronic syndrome is demonstrated by cognitive and behavioural changes which include apathy, psychomotor retardation, impaired memory and concentration.

The community mental health practitioner can play an important part in enabling the client to remain in their own home and maintain their independence. Full use of available resources specific to the client's needs is important and contact with local and national specialist agencies may be useful, for instance the Terence Higgins Trust or London Lighthouse, alongside liaison with local health specialists. Partners and relatives will also require support, advice and help to cope with the diagnosis and prognosis.

HOUSING

The discharge of clients from institutional care to the community is something which most professionals feel is intrinsically positive. However, it is vital that the housing and accommodation which is provided to discharged clients, or to people who are at risk of mental illness, is adequate in order to ensure that they are not at further risk from the housing itself. The core provision of housing, for people in the community with mental health problems, is similar to that for any other group. Individuals may live alone or with their families in their own homes. They may be able to live in public sector rented accommodation which is mostly provided by local councils. Given the current political climate, local authority provided housing is becoming less available, with housing often provided through housing associations. Problems may be experienced by clients wherever they live, but this is found particularly in relation to privately rented accommodation, where issues of exploitation and abuse of vulnerable clients have frequently been highlighted.

Clients with particular needs may need to have their accommodation adapted to take account of their situation. Staffed or supervised accommodation may be available for clients recently discharged from care in hospital, particularly if it is felt that they are vulnerable and would not be able to look after themselves properly. This may be either short term, as part of a process of rehabilitation leading to independent living in the near future, or it may be an alternative to hospital living for the client needing continuing care in a new setting. An alternative to ongoing care which is sometimes used is the provision of supported accommodation with families in the community, which can be very successful.

A number of issues relating to housing and accommodation for clients in the community may be of concern to the practitioner working with them.

The current moves to privatize social housing accommodation means that there is less direct influence on the part of local councils and politicians on this area than there once was. The responsibility for housing as part of planned care programmes cannot be discounted by the multidisciplinary team involved in community care. Clients living in accommodation alone may need active involvement in day care facilities that will not only reduce their social isolation, but also provide them with exposure to the social skills that they may well have left hospital without. Knowledge of local organizations and self-help groups is obviously vital in the continuing support particularly of clients whose accommodation is perceived by themselves or the practitioner to be contributing negatively to their mental health.

IMPLEMENTATION

Once goals have been identified and interventions that will achieve these goals have been planned, the practitioner can then start working with the client, and family where appropriate, on the implementation stage. It is important when implementing care in the community that all those involved in this process have a very clear idea of what is hoped to be achieved and what their part in it will be, so that the practitioner can rely on work carrying on in their absence and can receive feedback from a variety of sources that will help in the evaluation of progress. Time spent explaining the plan of care to all who will be involved in its implementation may seem unnecessary but it is invaluable in the long term, providing the family with information about the care that has been planned so that they can see the need for their involvement and also helping them to recognize potential areas that may give concern and need reporting. Feedback from the client and the family will also show whether the interventions are appropriate in practice or whether they need to be altered. Since the practitioner may only see the client once a fortnight, reassessment should be made of the progress of the client using these interventions on every occasion when they meet and the client encouraged to keep a written record of the work that is done and the results achieved during the absence of the practitioner.

The encouragement from the practitioner and relevant others will help to motivate the client during the times when he or she is not in direct contact with the practitioner. This provision of support and positive attitude maintenance is of particular importance when working in the community where the client could feel isolated and demotivated.

The utilization of all available resources should be considered in the implementation stage in order to avoid this risk as much as possible.

INDIVIDUAL PERFORMANCE REVIEW (*see also* Management supervision; Professional development)

This form of appraisal is often carried out formally on an annual basis rather than as an integral part of management supervision. The review should be a positive one, identifying what is to be done over the coming period, the barriers, past performance training needs and schedules designed to meet these requirements. The paperwork involved is merely the tool to assist in the process and this formalization of the process should not deter from the process itself. It is useful as a checklist and forms a record for both parties. For the process to succeed it is important that the employee own their objectives.

Preparation is necessary and the appraisee should have the opportunity to consider their performance, any changes necessary for the job, objectives and any barriers requiring resolution. Personal aims and development requirements should be identified. The manager should be prepared and experience a similar process. Confidentiality is important, as is the paperwork which ensures a record for future review and a systematic framework.

Performance review offers the opportunity to reflect upon job design, objective setting and training requirements. It offers the practitioner a chance of knowing how they are doing in their job and of identifying the goal posts for the future.

INFORMATION TECHNOLOGY

The single greatest challenge to practitioners has been the vastly increasing availability of collectable information. Clearly there is a need to pinpoint precisely what information should usefully be collected now and for the future. Community mental health practitioners have long been expected to record their daily activities and client contacts. In many areas this has been paper based, but as information technology develops this is increasingly being recorded via computer. Paper-based systems did not readily allow the exchange of clinical information or activity, between teams, departments, hospitals or the NHS. For the first time there is the opportunity, with the use of an appropriate coding system such as Read Version 3.00 and the necessary computer technology, for the NHS to produce integrated data analysis. Therefore the use of information technology in community mental health care has become part and parcel of the practitioner's role.

The use of information technology can be broadly divided into hardware and software components.

Hardware

Hardware is the term for the piece of physical equipment. These can vary from full size networked personal computers to miniature versions or hand-held computers, down to bar-code reading devices. Their use varies depending on the required function.

- Full-size network personal computers are used to exchange electronic mail, access client information systems, write case notes, letters and so on.
- Miniature version computers and hand-held computers are primarily designed with portability in mind; these are often used by practitioners in the field to record clinician activity and client contact information. They can often be as sophisticated as full-size computers.
- Bar-code reading devices are used to record clinician activity and client contact information. These are clearly less versatile and limited in their functionality.

Clearly a fully functioning network personal computer offers the greatest versatility in the use of software but is limited as it is not portable. Miniature computers are developing in sophistication and are beginning to be used with mobile phones to enable network connections to be made to hospitals, for instance, whilst in the field. However, currently the prohibitive cost of such systems appears to limit their usefulness. There is great diversity in the range of miniature computers, some of which now enable users to write on the screen as well as use the keyboard. Bar-code readers come in a variety of formats from the static laser design used by super-markets, through portable laser designs which can read bar-codes at a distance, to small pen-like devices which are 'swiped' across a printed code.

Software

Software can be defined as the instructions to a computer which make it function. This can range from the basic operating system through to specific application for word-processing, databases, spread-sheets and clinical information systems. Operating systems are currently in a state of transition. Microsoft products are a popular choice for many people purchasing software; this includes the Microsoft Windows operating system, which has recently upgraded to Windows 95. Generally full-size computers will use a version of the Microsoft Windows operating system, but in the miniature computer market there is a much wider range of operating systems. This can sometimes lead to difficulties in linking full-size computers and their information with hand-held computers. This particularly becomes an issue when practitioners are using client information systems.

Clinical information systems

Clinical information systems vary greatly in sophistication. At the most basic they provide a facility to record client admission and discharge information. The most sophisticated systems now offer practitioners the opportunity to record client needs, clinician activity and outcomes of care both in the office and whilst visiting clients.

Security

Administering a computer system requires care and attention. There are real threats to security of clinical information which come in a variety of forms. Physical destruction of computer equipment by fire, theft, or vandalism can occur. Network computer systems are vulnerable to 'hacking' (the unlawful access of information by an unauthorized person) and corruption of information by software viruses. The responsible system administrator will ensure that:

- local Trust policies are in place for the regular back-up of confidential information;
- staff training in the use of equipment and in the back-up of information is implemented;
- staff are trained to recognize the hazards of introducing unauthorized software to the computer systems.

A major consideration is accessibility to confidential clinical information. Only those people that are directly involved in a client's care should have access to clinical information relating to that individual.

Information technology is developing at an exponential rate, software is becoming more sophisticated, computers are becoming faster and communication between computers and networks is expanding. The ultimate expression of this is the Internet (the network of networks) which links thousands of computer networks throughout the world. Information technology can potentially herald an exciting and powerful development to clinical practice but at the same time the improved communication opportunities can be misused. Practitioners need to temper the greater opportunities presented with sensible practical precautions.

INSTITUTIONAL BEHAVIOUR

First described by Barton (1959) and Goffman (1961), this refers to behaviour commonly demonstrated by clients who have spent lengths of time in institutions. It happens as a result of routines imposed upon individuals which result in them losing the skills of social interaction. Dependence on the institution grows until the individual gradually loses interest and initiative, becoming passive and compliant and unable to take independent decisions.

With the closure of large mental institutions during the past few years, there are many clients in the community who may have been in hospital for years and who display this type of behaviour. The community practitioner is in an ideal position, among others, to attempt to restore independence to the optimum level possible for each client. Realistically, some clients may be so damaged by the effects of the institution that on leaving hospital they are unable to live independently and may spend the rest of their lives in supported accommodation. However, those less badly affected may be living in bed and breakfast accommodation or with their families.

Priority on working with clients who have spent years in hospital is an accurate assessment of their level of functioning in every sphere of their lives. For example: how do they manage money? What supports do they have? How do they spend their day? This assessment is a primary and continuing process and is accompanied by the formation of clear behaviourally structured stages to restore independence, employing all the resources at the practitioner's disposal. Involvement of the family in the process will be extremely helpful, particularly in terms of day-to-day monitoring of progress, since the evaluation of this progress will determine the next set of goals. However, be aware that any progress will be slow, depending on the level of institutional behaviour, and achievements may seem very small.

INTERVENTION STYLES (*see also* Communication and Relationship-building techniques)

Community mental health practitioners need to be aware of the way they relate to their clients. For most practitioners, a relationship forms the basis of the help and therapy they provide. Counselling and relationship-building skills may assist practitioners in understanding the content and context of their interactions but not necessarily an awareness of their own particular style or approach. John Heron (1986) has provided a usable guide to enable practitioners to assess and consider their interactions with clients. He suggests that all interactions may be classified into six broad categories, each of which has advantages and disadvantages to their use. It is the task of individual practitioners to examine their own interactions, to understand better what their preferences are and what best suits their clients. The interventions identified by Heron are either prescriptive or facilitative in style. Either is appropriate at the right time, but the over-use of either may be harmful.

Prescriptive interventions

These are seen to be directive to the client. They may involve meeting information needs, with the practitioner giving guidance such as 'I recommend you ...' or 'I think you should ...'.

Informative interventions are another form of prescriptive interventions which are less directive. They too are involved in providing information or instruction to the client. For instance, giving advice about how to take medication or catch a bus.

The third category of prescriptive intervention involves confronting interventions. These provide challenges to aspects of the client's behaviour. Together, these three may provide us with a framework to identify and understand the directive elements of interaction between community mental health practitioners and their clients.

Facilitative interventions

These involve practitioners in supporting rather than guiding their clients. They may be cathartic interventions that facilitate the release of emotions, draw clients out and encourage them to discuss issues further. Facilitative interventions may also involve supportive interventions which support, validate or encourage the client in some way. Heron's dimensions of facilitator style are an important tool enabling practitioners in the community to understand and identify the components of their interactions with their clients. Insight into one's own style makes for a safer practitioner. There will be times when the 'counsellor' **facilitates** 'client' independence, and other times when the 'nurse' **prescribes** 'patient' action. Practitioners using Heron's Six Category Intervention Analysis will discover whether their intervention style leans towards the prescriber or the facilitator. Ideally, the general approach should lie somewhere between the two with prescription or facilitation being used appropriately and with insight.

INTERVIEWS (*see also* Relationship-building skills; Assessment)

When an interview takes place in the practitioner's territory such as a clinic, the setting tends to be fairly formal. If a desk separates the practitioner from the client, this can set the scene for 'prescriber' action. This interview approach is structured to make best use of the time limitations of the appointment and enable the practitioner to gather specific information. When a counselling approach is used, more consideration is given to seating arrangements that facilitate spontaneity and partnership status. However, community mental health practitioners spend much of their working week interviewing clients and carers in a wide variety of settings where they have little or no control over the environment. The client may be in their own territory where they have more say in the proceedings, or the practitioner may visit the client in a day centre, ward, residential home or other location. Although practitioners are guests rather than hosts in these situations, they can still ensure that confidentiality and privacy are respected.

Unlike the clinic where the interviewer determines the environment, the home visit can involve many distractions. Pets leaping, telephones ringing and visitors calling can be frustrating if the interviewer wants to conduct a structured interview, but rewarding if the interviewer wants to observe the client's interactions and coping abilities. One advantage of undertaking interviews in the client's home is that the client can also be assessed on how they function in their own environment, and clues can be obtained about contributary factors to the client's problems.

In mental health counselling, the interview has many aims. During the initial interview practitioners will explain their role and begin to obtain the client's view of the referred problem. Some history-taking may take place but will not take priority over any emotional catharsis that occurs. If the client and a family member disagree over a problem then observation of how they interact and the roles each play might provide more helpful information at this initial stage than trying to intervene. The views expressed by family members and carers will help to complete the overall picture.

The building of a therapeutic relationship is facilitated during interviewing by the use of counselling skills. When a degree of trust has been established, practitioners can compare their assessment of the problem with client's or carer's views and begin the process of designing a care plan and a contract for its implementation. Once the initial interview has been carried out, an initial assessment will need to be forwarded to the referrer together with a plan of action. At subsequent interviews the aims may include: facilitating family communication, therapeutic intervention, monitoring and evaluation.

K

KNOWING YOUR PATCH

Mental health practitioners work in a multitude of different social and environmental settings and are able gradually to build up a complete picture of their catchment area. For the practitioner the local citizens' advice bureau, social services office, volunteer bureau or library are good starting points for seeking information. There are organizations specifically for carers' which can be local carer support groups or the larger organizations like Crossroads. The practitioner will discover that there is a charity organization for just about every disease and disability including Parkinson's, arthritis, diabetes, epilepsy, stroke and hearing impairment. Occasionally local papers publish a directory of useful organizations which list statutory services, that is mental health teams and clinics, local hospitals and day centres or non-statutory organizations including The Salvation Army, Samaritans, Relate, Cruse and Alcoholics Anonymous. If the information sought is related specifically to mental health resources then the practitioner's colleagues within the multidisciplinary mental health team, the local branch of MIND or National Schizophrenic Fellowship could provide answers.

If information about services for the elderly is required, the useful contacts are: the team specializing in the mental health of the elderly, the social services care managers and Age Concern. The social services are able to provide practitioners with lists of local residential, aftercare and nursing homes. A meeting with a social worker would provide much local knowledge about groups and clubs to which practitioners could refer their clients. Many clubs are organized by the Church, and there are opportunities for clients to become involved in church activities and voluntary work.

Practitioners new to their patch are likely to have been given a short period of induction and orientation. This usually consists of a couple of weeks spent meeting staff, visiting key agencies, and being driven around the neighbourhood by a colleague who no longer has constantly to refer to a road map. It probably takes at least six months of home visiting and liaison work for practitioners to feel confident that they know their patch.

Induction visits help the practitioner to know where the community agencies are and what they do, but it is when liaising on behalf of clients that the practitioner begins to understand the functioning of the 'network of care'.

L

LABELLING

J. and E. Cumming (1957) looked at the attitude of a community towards mental illness and learnt that one of the factors in the social rejection of the mentally ill was 'labelling'. This involves attaching to the individual a psychiatric diagnosis. This diagnosis or label would then serve to bring socially unpredictable or 'deviant' behaviour under the umbrella of illness, management and treatment, thus isolating individuals until they could be reintegrated into the community 'cured' and 'predictable'.

Crowcroft (1967) points out that labels can have a practical use, assisting in the organization and planning of mental health services and the assessing of future needs. Labels also enable us to consider what treatment facilities to offer people. Diagnostic labels are used when professionals discuss their clients' presentation of symptoms and behaviour. This form of professional jargon or short-hand may speed up communication but does not allow for the differences in the degree of illness or the behaviour presentations of the labelled condition. Unfortunately, labelling can also serve to keep the individual in the illness role whereby behaviour displayed may be assumed to be the product of the condition. Physical symptoms may be mistakenly labelled as psychosomatic and assertiveness may be labelled as unco-operative or aggressive behaviour. Social theorists Lemert (1967) and Scheff (1966) described how 'primary' deviant behaviour, seen by society as unusual or eccentric, resulted in the psychiatrist (acting for the community) labelling the individual as ill. Once labelled, the 'patient' begins to manifest additional behaviour abnormalities including the posturing, social withdrawal and apathy that Lemert described as 'secondary deviation' (Clare, 1976).

A vicious circle develops. Gradually the individual begins to adopt the label that has been applied, and behaves accordingly (Simmons and Brooker, 1986).

The mental health practitioner, with an insight into the advantages and disadvantages of labelling, is in a better position to assess an individual's problems within their social context and to see that some presentations of illness can be related to life problems rather than their diagnosis. Conversely, with more people willing to seek help from a mental health service that is more accessible, the risk of acquiring a psychiatric label for life problems may be greater (Simmons, 1986).

LEARNED HELPLESSNESS

First identified by Seligman (1975), this term refers to a state of impaired motivation, apathy, cynicism and withdrawal brought about when an individual feels that he no longer has control over his life. It is often apparent in those suffering from a long depressive illness who perceive that attempts to change their lives, or the feelings from which they are suffering, are futile. A vicious circle becomes established, where attempts inconsistent with personality or environment are seen to fail, thus reinforcing the belief that failure is inevitable. This reaction has to be gently challenged by the practitioner in a cognitive manner. It is important that the client is offered the opportunity to reframe the beliefs that have led to this condition and to see that thinking about their failure, with the support of the practitioner, can lead to a different approach. It may be useful to explore with clients factors that are hindering their behaviour and, on a more positive note, to look at the factors that may help them to change behaviours and achieve the goals that are seen as desirable.

LEGAL VULNERABILITY

Community mental health practitioners are particularly vulnerable with regard to the legal implications of their work. They care for a client group that can be unpredictable or irrational at times. In the community, the practitioner usually works alone, with no immediate supervision and with much autonomy. Practitioners often take on an advocacy role whereby their clients invest a high degree of trust and confidentiality in the relationship. As a consequence, practitioners can be open to a wide range of civil actions being brought against them. Allegations may be made against the practitioner that come under the following legal areas:

* negligence
* breach of confidentiality

- theft
- assault (violent or sexual).

In addition, practitioners should be aware of their vulnerability in other legal areas including:

- the misuse of drugs
- consent to treatment
- defamation of character.

Practitioners should also check their legal position in regard to carriage of drugs and the transporting of clients in practitioners' cars.

It is extremely important that practitioners have the cover of personal indemnity insurance. This can be obtained either through a professional organization, a union or an insurance broker. It is also advisable to check and adhere to service and team operational policies.

A good working knowledge of The Mental Health Act 1983 is essential for any community mental health practitioner.

LIFE EVENTS (*see also* Stress and coping)

Throughout an individual's life there are transitional stages requiring adjustments to previous routines and adaptation to the changes caused by life events. This tests the individual's coping mechanisms and can be both stressful and a challenge at the same time (Brown and Harris, 1978). Life events can be itemized under two broad headings.

Developmental

These life events may be foreseen as they are either part of physiological maturing or social customs.

Some examples are: adolescence, starting a first job, getting married, children leaving home and retirement.

Accidental

These life events are not foreseen and therefore the onset of stress can be more acute due to the fact that there is less time to prepare mentally for the adjustment required.

Some examples are: personal injury or illness, loss of a job, separation and bereavement.

Holmes and Rahe (1967) obtained average rankings from approximately 100 people of how stressful 43 events in a person's life are perceived to be. The death of a spouse proved to rank highest in stress value.

The stress associated with life events can be positive or negative. Such events as marriage, moving to a new house, going away on holiday and winning the lottery are usually viewed as positive events. Even so, they still involve adjusting to change and coping with the event.

In addition to the practical changes that have to be undergone, the individual also has to change the way he perceives himself and in the way he thinks and feels. Life events, positive or negative, create opportunity – the opportunity to increase one's armoury of coping mechanisms and, by the learning involved in coping with a new life event, to be better prepared to cope with the next.

Coping mechanisms can be adaptive or maladaptive. When adaptive it enables the person to cope in a healthy way. The mechanism allows the person to grow and develop with additional life skills. When maladaptive, the mechanism can result in the individual passing through the life event in an unhealthy way with the consequence that they will not make all the necessary adjustments required to enable them to move successfully forward.

During a life event, the individual may suffer a mental health problem and require psychiatric help to enable them to find the resources within themselves to cope and to learn from the experience. It is therefore essential for the practitioner to give much consideration to life events when assessing and history-taking.

When interviewing, practitioners should see individuals in the context of their family and social life. The individual is part of a family system and therefore a change in the individual will have an effect on the family system. Likewise, families also go through developmental and accidental life events and every family member is affected in some way by the changes.

MANAGEMENT SUPERVISION (*see also* Accountability; Clinical supervision; Individual performance review; Setting up supervision)

There is a need to supervise others managerially when working in a hierarchical structure and organization. The manager has a responsibility and duty to ensure that employees have management supervision. The amount of management supervision required is dependent upon the level of management function within the supervisees role. In management supervision the manager brings the agenda – the topics for discussion. Areas for discussion may include budgets, recruitment issues, development and resource issues and on some occasions caseload issues. In some organizations a form of clinical/management supervision has developed and also clinical/Individual Performance Review (IPR) developments. Strict guidelines as to the differences between these need to be assured at the outset.

Any manager should consider what management is and recognize the main components: 'running the business' and 'working with people' (Nelson, 1989). A more senior manager will be involved with the corporate strategic overview of running a business, whereas first level managers (those at the coalface) will be involved in organizing people dealing with immediate problems and the motivation of staff.

Managerial skills are required at all practitioner levels of an organization to ensure that the aims and objectives of the business are met. Common themes include the following.

1. **Organizational skills**: this involves ensuring that resources are used most effectively. The practitioner in the community organizes his time and visits according to distance, meetings, priority needs and so on.

2. **Role within the health care organization**: with the development of the internal market problems can be caused due to inconsistencies of roles amongst professionals. On occasions the aims of the profession may be dichotomous to those of the health care organization. This may cause conflict for the individual practitioner and affect their work, role, practice and relationships.
3. **Effective use of resources available**: it is necessary to recognize people's abilities and skills and use these effectively to ensure a high quality service to clients. All staff should be involved and contribute to service developments. This enables staff in being well-informed, trained, motivated and participating in their service.
4. **Responsibility**: managers are responsible for ensuring that policies, procedures, professional regulations and good practice managerially and professionally are implemented.

Wherever practice occurs levels of management also exist, so recognition that all practitioners have management skills is important. All practitioners should have access to and access management supervision. Business meetings may be available and occur on a group basis but appraisals/IPR should occur individually.

MANAGING MANIPULATION

The management of the client who is using manipulation poses considerable challenges to the practitioner working in the field of community mental health. Practitioners may need to ask themselves if the client is indeed manipulative or whether that label is being applied in an inappropriate way. Clients can and may be manipulative. However, the term may also indicate clients are seeking ways of managing the care being provided for them in a way that is different from the care planned by the professional. The client may be finding it difficult to challenge the practitioner openly or may be anxious about the consequences of expressing dissatisfaction or concern.

Attempts by clients to manipulate practitioners may take place, however, and it is important to recognize this and respond appropriately. A number of behaviours may be demonstrated by the client who is attempting to manipulate. Attempts at ingratiation may occur, involving a variety of behaviours on the client's part but characteristically indicating to the practitioner that he or she is 'special' or that 'nobody has ever cared for me so well before'. While this may be true and may reflect the client's experience, it could also be an attempt to create alliances between the client and the practitioner against other members of the multidisciplinary team. This is likely to have adverse consequences on the therapeutic relationship and needs to be addressed directly with the client, with the team and through supervision.

Aggression can be difficult to manage in a community setting. It is a very powerful tool by which a client may be able to manage the relationship with a practitioner. It is important that attempts at manipulation using aggression are handled firmly, though the safety of the practitioner and other people is clearly a major consideration in practical management. Openness and genuineness are vital qualities for the practitioner who is faced with manipulation. It is essential that any amendments to care plans are undertaken in conjunction with the rest of the multidisciplinary team and that they fit within the strategy of care which has been agreed. An open approach which allows the practitioner and client to be clear about apparent attempts at manipulation may result in positive change. Clinical supervision may also assist the practitioner to cope with the personal stress of working with this form of challenging behaviour. Responding to manipulation in the community setting is particularly challenging due to the practitioner working in relative therapeutic isolation. Support from colleagues is particularly necessary. A consistent, open and direct approach can minimize opportunities for manipulation to be used on the practitioner and maximize the possibility of effective therapeutic interventions and relationships.

MANIA (*see also* Depression)

The manic depressive disorders are characterized by disturbance of affect (i.e. mood). The mood may become elated or irritable (mania), or depressed (psychotic/endogenous depression). The disorder is usually recurrent, with episodes of depression or elation occurring on a cyclic basis. The term 'unipolar' is used for those clients who suffer repeated episodes of depression but do not experience mania, and the term 'bipolar' is used when clients experience alternating mania and depressive episodes. Manic or excited behaviour may also be seen in other disorders including schizophrenia, organic brain disease and in the effects of drugs such as amphetamines. The term 'hypomania' is used to describe the milder form of mania. Clients may be able to maintain a degree of control over their symptoms for brief periods and display some insight. The practitioner will observe evidence of increased physical activity and pressure of speech. Clients' moods can easily change from being euphoric and over-friendly to irritable and hostile and they may delight in informing the practitioner of plans for financial ventures that in reality are ill-conceived and beyond the client's means. Being easily distracted the client will quickly lose interest in one idea or train of thought and pursue another. When mania is 'moderate', the client may display grandiose and delusional ideas. Hostility may be more pronounced and aggression more likely. Sleep is often reduced with early waking and the commencement of early over-activity. There may be an increase in appetite with a corresponding reduction in manners and social skills. Libido may be increased and behavioural disinhibition may take place. Ideas can change so rapidly that it will be difficult for the practitioner to follow them (flight of ideas), and the client's insight is likely to be impaired. Severe or acute mania results in hyperactivity, bizarre and persecutory delusions and hallucinations. During episodes of mania clients can sometimes commit offences involving theft, fraud or, occasionally, violence. When undertaking an assessment, the practitioner will need to obtain a history from the carer as well as the client. Because the client is euphoric in mood there could be some denial of problems. The practitioner should bear in mind that disinhibited behaviour could also be the result of a cortical lesion or intoxication from drugs or alcohol. The assessment will also need to include judgements on the severity of the disorder, any causative factors, and the effects that the illness is having on both client and carers. Usually the causes of a manic disorder are largely endogenous but it is important to identify any life events that may have provoked the onset. Some cases follow physical illness, treatment by drugs (especially steroids), or operations (Gelder *et al.*, 1994). When the practitioner is involved in helping a client with a known history of hypomania and is able to intervene at an early stage, then it may be possible to treat and maintain the client in their own home. Support for both client and carer while ensuring compliance with medication may be enough to prevent exacerbation of the disorder from mild to a more severe mania. The client's euphoric mood, distractability and impaired insight can make counselling very difficult. Clients with a history of manic depressive psychosis are usually maintained on lithium as this tends to have prophylactic benefits in preventing or reducing the degree of cyclic mood swings. When a manic relapse seems to be imminent, then the major tranquillizers haloperidol or chlorpromazine tend to be prescribed, particularly when there is an acute episode. Unless the mania is mild, hospital admission is usually required to protect the client from the consequences of his own actions. Unfortunately, due to the client's lack of insight, poor treatment compliance, and euphoric or aggressive mood, compulsory admission is often needed. Following an episode of mania, the practitioner will have to re-establish the previous rapport that is likely to have been strained by the event. This can be made more difficult if compulsory hospitalization was instigated. Keeping the client well will require a dual medical and psychosocial approach. The importance of adhering to the prescribed medication must be emphasized, with the practitioner encouraging compliance, monitoring the effects of medication, and arranging for regular lithium tests to be undertaken. In addition to the practitioner's home visits, outpatient follow-up and/or day hospital support can also be arranged. Mania is regarded by some to be a defence mechanism against depression. It is common for manic clients to lapse into depression quite rapidly and the practitioner will need to be vigilant for this. It is very stressful for families caring for relatives suffering repeated episodes of mania, and practitioners will find themselves working very closely with carers in these situations. Often, practitioners provide this support over many years, with the advantage of being alerted at a very early stage when the illness shows signs of recurring.

MEDICATION AND MENTAL HEALTH (*see also* Side effects of medication; Anxiety management)

The use of drugs in treating mental illness is commonplace and will often run concurrently with other therapeutic approaches. Mental health practitioners in the community will need to be aware of their client's prescribed medications and consider both the therapeutic and adverse effects of these in the overall treatment plan.

The community psychiatric nurse (CPN) has an important role to play in the administration and monitoring of psychotrophic drugs and is also well placed to liaise between the client, the GP and the psychiatrist. There are various avenues for the prescribing of these drugs. The client's GP may prescribe them without reference to the psychiatrist and refer directly to the CPN for monitoring to ensure that the medication is taken correctly and is having the desired effect. Alternatively, the client may receive their first prescription while in hospital and, when discharged, continue with the medication with repeat prescriptions from their GP. The psychotrophic medication can be reviewed by the psychiatrist in the psychiatric outpatient clinic and the CPN is able to facilitate communication to see that cross-prescribing does not occur.

A regular CPN visit to the client's home has many advantages. Such visits can ensure that the client's ability to cope with daily tasks is not impaired by drug intolerance or side effects such as drowsiness. The CPN is able to explain what the drugs are for and to reassure the client about any concerns they may have about them. In addition, the CPN can obtain the views of the informal carers regarding the client's progress on the medication. The CPN is able to encourage and reassure where there is a tendency to non-compliance as is sometimes the case when depot injections are administered. Monitoring correct dosages and the removal of excess tablets is particularly important where there is a risk of suicide. The CPN also has a role in monitoring the mental state and mood of the client who is on lithium carbonate and in ensuring that regular tests are undertaken to maintain the correct blood lithium level. Conversely, a CPN may be involved in overseeing a tranquillizer withdrawal programme and complement this with the teaching of anxiety management and relaxation techniques.

MENTAL HEALTH ACT 1983 (*see also* Mental Health Act Code of Practice)

Introduction

The provisions of The Mental Health Act 1983 relate predominantly to achieving compulsory admission to hospital and the care and treatment of clients thus detained. There are however some sections of The Mental Health Act with particular relevance for community mental health nurses. The most significant is section 117 which relates to aftercare, but community mental health nurses should also have a working knowledge of admission sections (sections 2, 3, 4, 135 and 136) which will be needed from time to time for clients already on their caseload.

Assessment for admission

Sections 2 and 3 are the most commonly used and both are founded on two medical recommendations accompanied by an application for admission made by an approved social worker (ASW). Section 2 is an assessment section allowing detention for up to 28 days, section 3 is a treatment section allowing detention and treatment for up to six months. The decision as to which section to use is made by the ASW and the doctors on the basis of the history and assessment. One of the medical recommendations must be made by a doctor approved under section 12 of the Act. Additionally, if practicable, one of the recommendations should be made by a doctor with previous knowledge of the client. The ideal choice, therefore, would be the consultant and the client's GP. The ASW has overall responsibility for co-ordination of the assessment and good practice would include a discussion with the community mental health nurse on events preceding the request for an assessment.

Where the ASW considers admission to be an urgent necessity and there is a delay obtaining a second medical recommendation the ASW may arrange an emergency admission under section 4 on the basis of a single medical recommendation.

Section 136 is the police power to remove a person found in a public place and thought to be suffering from a mental illness to a place of safety.

Section 135 is the warrant issued by a justice of the peace to search for and remove a person thought to be suffering from a mental illness to a place of safety. Under this section the police can gain access to a person in their home by forcible entry if necessary. The ASW is responsible for applying to the justice of the peace for the warrant.

If, on the basis of a visit to a patient or a report from relatives, friends or neighbours, a community mental health nurse suspects a Mental Health Act assessment is needed this should be reported to the appropriate ASW, the client's GP and the consultant psychiatrist; in exceptional circumstances it may also be necessary to involve the police.

Aftercare

Section 117 requires district health authorities and local social services to provide aftercare to people who have been detained under sections 3, 37, 47 and 48.

Chapter 27 of the *Code of Practice for The Mental Health Act* (DoH, 1993a) describes the purpose of aftercare as enabling a patient to return to his home and to minimize the chance of his needing future inpatient hospital care. This is to be achieved through multiprofessional clinical meetings which will devise a care plan to meet the client's continuing health and social care needs.

In many instances the person appointed as keyworker will be a community mental health nurse. The main responsibilities of the keyworker are to ensure that the care is delivered as planned and to arrange regular reviews of the plan. Where the community mental health nurse is also providing a significant proportion of the care the monitoring task will be less onerous; however, the amount of time needed for liaison and administration should not be underestimated.

MENTAL HEALTH ACT CODE OF PRACTICE (*see also* The Mental Health Act 1983)

The first edition of the *Code of Practice* was published in 1990 and the second edition was published in 1993 (DoH, 1993). The *Code of Practice* provides practical guidance on the application of The Mental Health Act 1983 but does not carry legal powers in itself.

> The Act does not impose a legal duty to comply with the Code but failure to follow the Code could be referred to in evidence in legal proceedings (DoH, 1993, page 1).

The vast majority of guidance on the *Code of Practice* relates to the process of admission to hospital under the Mental Health Act, assessment and treatment while detained in hospital and the client's rights throughout this process. The two sections of greatest interest to community mental health nurses are assessment prior to possible admission under The Mental Health Act and leaving hospital. Community mental health nurses are mentioned explicitly in sections 2.16, 2.26 and 2.28.

Section 2.16 relates to the responsibilities of the social worker and states:

> The ASW (approved social worker) should consult wherever possible with other professionals who have been involved in the patient's

care, for example home care staff or community psychiatric nurses (CPNs).

Section 2.26 relates to medical responsibilities and states:

It is particularly important that any CPN concerned with a patient's care be fully involved in the taking of such a decision.

The decision referred to in this quotation is referral to other agencies or services when admission is felt not to be appropriate.

Section 2.28 relates to disagreements between the ASW and medical staff and states:

Sometimes there will be differences of opinion between assessing professionals. There is nothing wrong with disagreements: handled properly these offer an opportunity to safeguard the interest of the patient by widening the discussion on the best way of meeting the patient's needs. Doctors and the ASWs should be ready to consult colleagues (especially CPNs and other community care staff involved with the patient's care), while retaining for themselves the final responsibility.

These brief references to the role of the community mental health nurse grossly understate the importance of the detailed knowledge they have of clients on their caseload. Throughout the section on assessment doctors and social workers are required to refer to evidence of the client's behaviour, mental state and psychiatric history. The community mental health nurse will often be the person with the most detailed and objective information and should therefore be consulted throughout the process of assessment.

Individuals detained under sections 3 and 37 of The Mental Health Act are entitled to aftercare under section 117 of the Act. In the vast majority of cases the person responsible for the delivery and coordination of this aftercare will be a community mental health nurse. The principles of section 117 have been extended to all individuals being discharged from psychiatric hospitals and others being accepted for care in the community through the Care Programme Approach. The specific requirement of section 117 is that the responsible medical officer (RMO) should convene a case conference prior to the client's discharge which will be attended by all relevant professionals and agencies who will be involved in the client's aftercare. It is at this meeting that the keyworker will be appointed and any community mental health nurse attending such a meeting should ensure that they are absolutely clear at the end of the meeting whether or not they have been appointed to this role. Such decisions are often made by default which can lead to serious disruption of the delivery of aftercare.

The introduction to the *Code of Practice* describes the broad principles of how individuals subject to The Mental Health Act should be treated. They are as follows.

1.3 The Code provides much detailed guidance, but this needs to be read in the light of the following broad principles, that people being assessed for possible admission under the Act or to whom the Act applies should:
- receive respect for and consideration of their individual qualities and diverse backgrounds – social, cultural, ethnic and religious;
- have their needs taken fully into account though it is recognized that, within available resources, and may not always be practicable to meet them;
- be delivered any necessary treatment or care in the least controlled and segregated facilities practicable;
- be treated or cared for in such a way that promotes to the greatest practicable degree, their self-determination and personal responsibility consistent with their needs and wishes;
- be discharged from any order under the Act to which they are subject immediately it is no longer necessary.

These principles can and should be applied to all patients on a community mental health nurse's caseload and not just those subject to section 117 of The Mental Health Act.

MENTAL HEALTH BILL 1995

The Mental Health (Patients in the Community) Bill 1995 is the most recent initiative by the Government to ensure that people who are considered 'high risk' receive 'aftercare under supervision'.

It seeks to provide care for those people 16 years and over who have required hospital detention for treatment under section 117 of The Mental Health Act 1983, and on discharge are thought to be a risk to self, others or at risk of exploitation.

A care plan is arranged on discharge stating the need for the client to reside in a specific place, attend for treatment, occupation, education and training at specified times (Harrison, 1995). Failure to comply with these requirements can result in the nominated supervisor or anyone else they authorize to have the power to convey the client to the place or service identified in the care plan or convey them back to hospital (Dean, 1995). The Bill cannot force the client to receive treatment and the nominated supervisor (any member of the health care team) has no powers to enter the client's place of residence forcibly. The Bill is an addition to the current supervision registers which were developed for those people suffering from a severe mental illness who meet a similar criteria to that of The Mental Health Bill.

Both these initiatives intend to secure resources from the Departments of Health and Social Services and to ensure the person subject to aftercare under supervision, receives these.

An application for aftercare supervision is made to the health authority by the responsible medical officer (RMO) and is accompanied by written recommendations from the community responsible medical officer (who does not need to be section 12 approved but is responsible for medical aftercare) and an approved social worker (ASW). The criteria used for the application is:

1. the patient is suffering from a mental disorder;
2. substantial risk of serious harm to the health of the patient or the safety of other persons at serious risk of being exploited if aftercare services were not provided (Harrison, 1995).

Prior to making the application the RMO will consult with the client, a professional involved with treatment whilst an inpatient, a professional involved in aftercare and a significant other, for instance a carer who is not professionally qualified but is involved in aftercare.

The supervision order lasts for six months and can be renewed for a further period of six months and at subsequent yearly intervals subject to the above criteria being satisfied. The patient has the right of appeal to the Mental Health Review Tribunal (MHRT). Supervised aftercare ceases on the instructions of the RMO, MHRT, if the client is in custody, admitted to hospital under section or received into guardianship.

The Bill also allows the period of leave of absence to be extended from six months to one year and allows patients who have absconded for more than 28 days to be recalled to the hospital.

MENTAL HEALTH PROMOTION

Health promotion is an important role for community mental health practitioners. Traditionally those doing a nursing job in the community have been seen as 'doers' rather than as partners of the clients in their care. The public image is still very often that of the dependent person in the bed rather than the image of the potentially much more independent person in the community (UKCC, 1986).

The role of the health practitioner as a promoter of health, rather than just a carer of the ill, has never been greater. This is reinforced by the World Health Organization (with its *Health for All by the year 2000* (WHO, 1981) and the UK Government with its targets for the 'health of the nation' (DoH, 1995). It is clearly part of the role of those practitioners caring for clients with mental health problems to address how to avoid illness striking or, at least, to minimize the consequences when it does. Mental health promotion in practice will involve health education and preventative psychiatry. Preventative psychiatry and the model of 'Primary, Secondary, and Tertiary Prevention' has been well documented since Gerald Caplan's books were published in the 1960s and clearly demonstrate areas where mental health promotion and education can take place.

Primary prevention

Primary prevention aims to raise public awareness about mental health to reduce stigma and negative attitudes and to reduce the chances of people becoming mentally ill by better understanding of the causes.

Secondary prevention

Secondary prevention aims to minimize the effects of mental illness and provides early intervention to reduce the duration and severity of the illness.

Tertiary prevention

Tertiary prevention aims to reduce the residual effects of mental illness and the disabilities it leaves.

Health promotion at a primary level will involve the practitioner in giving health educational input to various social groups, including schools, residential homes, day centres, community centres, church groups, carer support groups and self-help groups. At a secondary level health promotion and education will take place mainly in the following areas.

1. Direct support and advice for individual clients and their informal carers.
2. Imparting knowledge and advice to the formal carers in the community, including the primary health care team, the social services and the private and voluntary sectors.
3. Facilitating group therapy work where clients are given the skills and knowledge to cope with their problems in a more independent way, for instance by using new social skills and anxiety management techniques.

When carrying out tertiary care, the practitioner will be working with clients who require long-term support and supervision. Many of these clients will have spent some years being cared for in the large psychiatric hospitals prior to rehabilitation into the community. Health promotion will be aimed at maintaining the client's optimal level of functioning on both a personal and social level, and supporting and advising those caring for them in the community. These carers may be the client's family or the care staff of aftercare homes.

The English National Board (1989), in a learning package on the subject of health promotion, sees key themes which influence the effectiveness of health promotion in the community. They seem to have relevance to all areas of practice. The focus of activity should be the client, not some abstract target or objective. It is also felt that there is a need for a partnership between the client and the practitioner, acknowledging what each is bringing to the relationship and recognizing the diversity of views which may exist.

This is in direct contrast to attempts to impose the professional's view on the client. In addition, it is suggested that groups are often helpful, especially for people who may be isolated in the community, as these allow sharing and mutual learning to take place.

MOTHER AND BABY – POSTNATAL MENTAL HEALTH NEEDS

The community mental health practitioner may come into contact with new mothers who have a mental illness. The mental distress may be following the birth of the child or present prior to the child's birth. There are three main types of psychological disorder associated with the puerperium. These are:

1. baby blues
2. postnatal depression
3. postnatal psychosis (puerperal psychosis).

As suggested, baby blues commonly occur around the third day following the birth of the baby and last a day or two. Postnatal depression occurs across all cultures and social classes. Kumar (1984) estimates that a degree of depression may arise in as many as one in ten mothers. The depression can last for several weeks or months. Consideration that the mother may be reluctant to seek help at this normally joyous time should be made. Puerperal psychosis is a more severe form of psychological disturbance and again is not related to any one culture or social group. Inpatient care may be necessary and it is important that facilities should be offered for both the mother and baby. Some acute psychiatric wards have mother and baby beds, but generally these are specialist regional units. Rating scales such as the Bethlem Mother–Infant Interaction Scale and the Edinburgh Postnatal Depression Rating Scales can be used for base-line measurement and assessment.

Care in the community setting for mothers with mental health illness may be through their health visitor, GP and community mental health nurse, but mainly the primary health care team. In some areas there are specialist community mental health wards and they would carry a caseload and offer expert advice and consultancy. Support groups and self-help groups are often used to offer support to women experiencing postnatal illness.

Mothers who have a mental illness prior to their pregnancy should require support and monitoring throughout their pregnancy especially with regards to any medication being taken. The community mental health practitioner is well placed to assist and support this group of patients.

MULTIDISCIPLINARY TEAMS

With the growth in community care in mental health, and the closure of the large psychiatric hospitals, multidisciplinary teams have been encouraged as the most effective method of providing care to clients with a wide range of needs that are inappropriately met by the traditional medical model approach to care. However, true multidisciplinary team **working** may be difficult to see in reality. This may be due to practitioners holding on to their traditional roles, or to the perpetuation of the medical model which emphasizes the hierarchy headed by a consultant. However, neither of these reasons are beneficial to the clients, since it makes more sense to combine the expertise available from a wide range of professional backgrounds in order to provide a comprehensive plan of care for the client. The team may consist of doctors, nurses, social workers, occupational therapists and psychologists, all of whom may have different ideas of how the team should operate. For example, Ovreteit (1993) sees four types of teams which have different methods of organization, ranging from the team which has a designated team manager to a team which runs on a democratic basis with no formal leader. While it is in a sense unimportant which model of organization is used, it is clearly vital that all the members of the team both agree with it and are quite clear of the individual roles of everyone in the team. Communication about the skills that each person has is also important, so that these individual areas of expertise can be recognized and utilized, and to avoid the understandable feelings of anxiety about being undervalued or disregarded in terms of professional development. Careful discussion of these points on a regular basis will help to avoid any tension between team members and enable the allocation of care for the client to the person(s) most able to provide it to the total benefit of the client.

NORMALIZATION – SOCIAL ROLE VALORIZATION

Normalization, as a concept, developed in Scandinavia and the North American continent throughout the 1950s, 60s and 70s. It is a philosophy which, its supporters claim, should be used to shape services for devalued people such as people with mental illness and learning disabilities (Nirje, 1969; Bank-Mikkelson, 1970). The origins of this philosophy can be traced to the raised awareness of human rights following the widespread abuse of human rights during the Second World War, and the work of many authors on the inhumane treatment meted out to the inmates of the long stay institutions for the 'mentally ill and handicapped' (Barton, 1959; Goffman, 1961).

One of the theorists most closely associated with the philosophy, Wolf Wolfensberger, developed this philosophy further throughout the 70s and 80s, and advocated the use of this approach in all human services (Wolfensberger, 1972).

Nirje (1969) defined normalization thus:

Normalization is the making available to the 'mentally retarded' patterns and conditions of everyday life which are as close as possible to the norms and patterns of the mainstream of society. An ordinary life includes a normal rhythm of days, weeks and years, normal-sized living units, adequate privacy, normal access to social, emotional and sexual relationships with others, normal growing up experiences, the possibility of decently paid work, choice and participation in decisions affecting one's work.

There was some criticism of the approach arising from misunderstandings over the use and meaning of the words 'normal' and 'ordinary': what is ordinary and normal is difficult to define and this approach could end as another attempt to impose certain lifestyles on users of a service. There were also examples of the rigid and zealous misapplication of normalization, which ran counter to the spirit of the philosophy (Mesibov, 1990; Gilbert, 1993).

As a result of these types of criticism, Wolfensberger developed the concept and redefined normalization as Social Role Valorization (Wolfensberger, 1983). This was an attempt to replace the concept of 'normality' and to focus on the real goal of services, which was to restore or add the positive social value which devalued people had been deprived of or denied. An example of this approach is that one is often socially judged by the company one keeps. If a person with mental illness is enabled to associate socially with other people of high social value, they in turn will be given a higher social value than they otherwise would have been given.

Again more recently, John O'Brien (1987) has developed the idea of the Five Service Accomplishments. O'Brien suggests that these service accomplishments should be the goals which practitioners should be striving to achieve for their clients. Moreover, rather than being just a set of goals, these accomplishments can also be used as a quality assurance tool. Services can be evaluated to determine the extent to which each of them is being met.

The Five Service Accomplishments

1. **Presence**: this is the extent to which an individual is able and encouraged to use resources and facilities used by the rest of the local community. For example, clients with mental illness or learning disabilities should use wherever possible, local GPs and other health and social services, shops, leisure and work facilities.
2. **Participation**: clients should not only have a visible presence in their local community but should be active within it, through participation in some of the various social activities enjoyed by the rest of the local population, in effect to be citizens. Examples of such participation could include being employees, participation in the running of their own homes and services, and perhaps ultimately to be active politically, through voting, lobbying and as elected representatives.
3. **Respect**: this is the extent to which clients are afforded respect and dignity, or given opportunities to gain it through achievement. Examples of this accomplishment are being treated and addressed as individuals, the avoidance of the use of degrading labels and the use of resources which mark an individual or group out as being 'abnormal' or different. The offering of first rate or high quality services is an example of recognition of this accomplishment.

4. **Choice**: this is the offering of a broad range of real choices to clients. It should always be more than 'a take it or leave it' approach, which for people with few options, is no choice at all. Instead, a variety of realistic choices should be offered and every opportunity should be given for clients to be involved in decision making. However, some clients who have been long-term clients of devaluing service may have lost confidence, either in their own decision making or that their choices will be respected. Therefore, practitioners must demonstrate their commitment to respecting and welcoming client choice.

5. **Competence**: this is the commitment of practitioners to teach meaningful skills to clients, so that they may develop the competence to become full citizens wherever possible, but which will also enhance other peoples' views of them. An example of the skill which clients should be given every chance to develop competence in is the means of self-expression. It is only through developing communication skills that someone can become self-determining. Assertiveness, self-care and other social skills are examples of the personal competence which will help restore value to the client, not just in their own eyes but in the view of others, who in the past may not have recognized that value.

O'Brien's framework has been used widely to develop services which are more person valuing, and adhere to the spirit of the original philosophy of normalization. Perhaps the real value of this approach is that it leaves scope for creativity and inventiveness; it allows the service provider to be original in the way in which these service accomplishments are achieved. It is this openness and lack of rigidity, as well as the scope for the inclusion of service users in making these sorts of decisions, which provide a useful way forward for developing and implementing this service philosophy.

NON-VERBAL COMMUNICATION

Individuals communicate not only verbally but also by the use of non-verbal communication in the form of body posture, gestures and eye contact. Non-verbal communication is usually considered to be a more accurate expression of an individual's feelings as people have less conscious control over non-verbal behaviour. From the initial meeting with a client the practitioner will cultivate a deliberate awareness of non-verbal communication. This involves using all of the senses to engage in a process identified by many authors as being 'active listening'. This includes observation skills, and being sensitive to covert verbal cues and messages. When listening, the practitioner not only hears the words communicated by the client but also observes the tone used and the accompanying expressions and gestures. The practitioner has to listen for other messages beneath the client's self-reporting, and be aware of any defences revealed by body language.

Observations can be made for any incongruity between what is being communicated verbally and non-verbally. Do the words say one thing and the clenched fist another? Does the client look out of the window or raise their eyes to the ceiling every time their partner speaks? Gestures, facial expressions and seating posture can reveal the client's agreement, frustration or anxieties in response to the practitioner's questions, paraphrasing or interpretations.

People interact non-verbally in a range of different ways. Lack of eye contact may indicate an individual with limited self-confidence. It may also be related to cultural expectations about dominance and subordinate relationships, or, simply, to individual styles of functioning. Similarly, variations in the acceptability of touch or another person sitting in close proximity may be of significance in revealing anxieties but they may also result from socialization and cultural expectations. In people's homes it is vital that the practitioner is sensitive to such variations and is able both to interpret and use non-verbal communication to enhance the interaction with their clients. Conversely, the practitioner's verbal and non-verbal behaviour will communicate to the client confirmation of active listening, genuine interest, empathy and respect. The client, consciously or unconsciously, will respond to the subtle non-verbal cues that the practitioner brings to the interview.

O

OBSERVATION AND MONITORING (*see also* Assessment)

Observation is best defined as 'a systematic gathering and recording of all the necessary information about a patient relevant to the production and monitoring of his nursing intervention and medical treatment' (Ward, 1985 page 10). Central to the planning of nursing care, observation is used as a foundation for assessment and the planning of interventions that will benefit the client. The main source of information gained is obviously the client but carers and other members of the team will also be able to provide their own views. Observation is based on objective criteria, not assumptions or subjective feelings that may arise during the relationship. Clients can be encouraged to record their own observations of their physical and mental state, using a previously agreed set of measures. These can take into account every facet of daily life, or can be a brief overview of one aspect of behaviour. The practitioner similarly may choose to observe in order to gain a total view of the client, or at times will focus on one particular aspect of the life of the client. Thorough observation is also important in the monitoring of the client's health and welfare and can lead to changes in the care that is given or planned.

OBSTACLES

The therapeutic process involved in working with clients in their homes can be blocked by what may seem small issues, but which can prevent a free flow of communication. Practitioners are faced with the knowledge that they are not on home ground, and that any attempt to minimize these obstacles must be made sensitively. Firstly, it is not uncommon to arrive at the client's house to discover that the television is a permanent loud and live feature of the living room. A tentative request for the television to be turned off often results merely in a turning down of the volume, with the images on the screen still serving as a distraction. Obviously, there is no wish to offend the client, yet the practitioner can be assertive by stating the need for concentration on the part of both the client and the practitioner on the important issues that may be discussed, and that this can best be achieved without the distraction of the television. Even this overt approach may fail and the practitioner is then faced with the difficult task not only of concentrating fully on the client, but of engaging the client in a relationship that is absorbing enough to 'tune out' the television.

The second obstacle, which is even more difficult to handle but which if left can create chaos, is the presence in the living room of one or more small children, who need attention and often resent the presence of the practitioner who is seen as an intruder. It may be unrealistic to expect that the parent can be seen in a room away from the children, or at a time when the children are not in the house, and here the practitioner has to utilize patience and persistent active listening skills. The crafty practitioner may just 'happen to have' a supply of felt tip pens and scrap paper which may achieve temporary peace. Hopefully, the practitioner can also discuss the problem with the client to see whether any compromise can be reached, since the client may be equally distracted by the presence of children and the subsequent lack of privacy.

Finally, dogs! The constant barking, and attempted 'nips' from a small dog can be quite distracting enough but, on a more serious note, the presence of a large dog which appears unfriendly and hostile can be very intimidating, and does not help the practitioner to feel relaxed. In this instance, the practitioner should inform the client of their feelings about the presence of the dog and request that it is removed from the room while the interview takes place. Most clients, when realizing that the practitioner is feeling unhappy or unsafe, will usually be prepared to shut the dog in the kitchen or garden for the duration of the visit.

In all these cases, it is evident that the interpersonal skills of the practitioner will be of paramount importance, firstly to avoid offending the client and secondly to ensure the growth of a helping relationship without, or in spite of, these obstacles.

OUTCOMES OF CARE

Caring for people with mental health problems in the community often involves a number of skilled health care professionals and lay carers. Questions are asked as to the value of the contributions from all involved in terms of cost, effectiveness and the nature of the work (Burdick *et al.*, 1994). It is argued that comparing similar cases and results in relation to the effectiveness of interventions on the client, themes can be identified and cost effective care delivered (Sale, 1991).

It is essential that all members of the team understand what the outcome of treatment is, what will the end result be and how the care that is delivered by individuals within the team will contribute to the health of the client. Outcomes generally refer to the impact of interventions on the client's health, welfare or satisfaction with the experience of care (Donabedian, 1980).

To establish how effective a practitioner and their interventions are requires the collection of data. This can be achieved by using question-naires, interviews, documentation, reviews, comparison of patient profiles, observation and the use of rating scales. A framework for systematically reviewing and analysing the data collected will need to occur in order to identify best practice.

PATIENT OR CLIENT? (*see also* Relationship-building skills; Empowerment)

Current community practitioners are more likely to be using the term client than patient for individuals receiving care in the community. With the advent of community care, practitioners were able to observe and support individuals within the context of family and social systems. Mental illness came to be viewed, in part at least, as problems of living or coping difficulties that may be the result of such factors as isolation, deprivation, relationship stresses or social skills deficits. The helping process began to move from curing the passive patient to enabling the individual to solve their problems within the context of a therapeutic relationship.

Simmons and Brooker (1986) remind us of principles underpinning community care such as:

- care based on individual need;
- the promotion of self-determination;
- minimal dependence;
- the individual's right to make choices.

These principles, when applied, would facilitate empowerment rather the passivity on the part of the individual receiving care. *The Concise Oxford Dictionary* defines 'patient' as 'a person receiving medical treatment'; 'client' is defined as 'a person using the services of a lawyer, architect, social worker or other professional person'. The client 'using' as opposed to the patient 'receiving', seems to suggest a more active role in the process. The use of the term client rather than patient reflects the more equal relationship between the providers and the users of services where much of the care and treatment is provided away from the practitioner's base and often in the client's home (Simmons and Brooker, 1986). Mental health practice that focuses on problem solving rather than illness, and a partnership model of care, will enable the individual to learn coping strategies. This will better equip the individual to cope with future crises as successful resolution of problems will lie with the client not with the prescriber.

PATIENT'S CHARTER

The Patient's Charter (2nd edn) (DoH, 1995) is generic in that it applies to all patients of the NHS. Although many of the sections apply to health care *per se*, a number are specific to mental health care.

The booklet is split into sections covering rights and standards through-out the NHS, GP services, hospital services, community services, ambulance services, dental, optical and pharmaceutical services. The following apply to mental health clients.

1. Clients can expect all the staff they meet face to face to wear name badges.
2. Clients can expect a qualified nurse, midwife or health visitor to be responsible for their nursing or midwifery care. They will be told the practitioner's name.

Re: community nurses

3. If a home visit is required clients can *expect* to be consulted about a convenient time. They can expect a visit within a two-hour band.
4. In exceptional circumstances, if the appointment is delayed or is cancelled, then the client should be informed and another re-arranged as soon as possible.
5. Clients can expect to receive a visit from a mental health nurse:

    (a) within four hours (in the daytime) if they have been referred to the practitioner as an urgent client;
    (b) within two working days, if referred as a non-urgent client and the practitioner is not asked to see them on a particular day;
    (c) By appointment on the day the client asks for if they give more than 48 hours notice.

Local community care charters are being developed with local authorities to cater for the standards of service expected from the increasing number of home care services.

A patient's charter specifically for mental health clients is also being discussed and developed.

PROBLEM SOLVING PROCESS

The principles of the nursing process are well established within mental health nursing. However, the practice of undertaking the process of assessment, planning, intervention and evaluation varies widely within community care. One important point to be made is the non-linear nature of the care process within the community. Information is not always acquired in the order in which it may be needed or relevant. The practitioner working in the community may need to accept that they will not always have all of the information which is needed to allow a full assessment to be undertaken prior to having demands for intervention made of them. The process needs to reflect the realities of care in the community, where the professional doesn't always hold all of the 'cards' in a relationship. A client's needs and views must be taken fully into account when information gathering, involving the client (and if necessary and permitted, family or significant others) in the vital task of assessment. It is also important to remember there may be access to a range of sources of information which is available in the community, which may assist the professional in gathering information. It may be considered that a failure by the practitioner to prepare themselves properly with information is a serious professional deficit. It is vital that information is understood and used appropriately.

The planning and implementation stages of the nursing process in the community must also be seen as clearly client centred. Failure to involve the client in their care, except in the most exceptional circumstances, must be seen as setting the community practitioner up to fail. Unless the care is owned by and agreed with the client, it is unlikely to be implemented effectively.

One of the weakest areas of the nursing process generally tends to be the fourth stage, evaluation. As with the previous stages, client involvement is central to the success of evaluation, which is itself of key importance to the problem solving cycle (or nursing process). The client's objectives also need to be considered, and should match the objectives set as part of the problem solving approach by the practitioner and client together. This is clearly good practice for all mental health practitioners. In the community, it is vital.

The problem solving cycle or nursing process is clearly central to good community care. In conjunction with selected conceptual frameworks the process provides the professional practitioner with a client centred and problem focused approach to care. Without this, client care is difficult to organize effectively.

PROFESSIONAL DEVELOPMENT (*see also* Individual performance review)

The client or user of any community mental health service is entitled to have care which is based upon knowledge and understanding of their specific mental health requirements. The mental health practitioner will need to be up to date with specific government initiatives, professional initiatives and local initiatives relating to this client group. This can be achieved through localized training set up within the employing organization, further study at higher education college or advertised study days.

In nursing there is a requirement that knowledge and theory applied to practice is updated. This is demonstrated through the compilation of a personal professional portfolio which will incorporate either information gained through study days or personal study and its application to practice. Over a period of three years, five days' study should be demonstrated. The English National Board advocates that nursing is about lifelong learning, rather than a training which obviates the need for any further gain of knowledge. The acknowledgement of this by nurses can be seen in the growing numbers of those enrolling either for the English National Board Higher Award or for post-registration studies.

Other disciplines within the multidisciplinary community mental health team may not have the same mandatory professional development, but strongly support the need for continuing professional development. This is not only for the benefit of clients and the provision of services, but also for career progression; there are increasing opportunities for professionals to undertake courses at Master's level in their professional field.

PROJECTION

The business of mental health care in the community is complicated somewhat by clients' use of mental or ego defence mechanisms. These relatively or absolutely unconscious mechanisms act to protect individuals from responses which they can't cope with, by allowing them to divert or change the response they would (unconsciously) like to make, to one which is more socially acceptable. The mechanism of projection is one of these.

Typically, it is reported as the mechanism which is deployed on return from a busy day's work, stressed and ready to mug the boss; instead, using projection, the approach taken by most of us is to take our frustrations out often on the person nearest to us.

With clients and carers using projection, the professional working in the community may find themselves on the receiving end of the process of projection. Moving into the client's home, the practitioner needs to be aware of the possibility of anger being directed at them which they don't necessarily deserve. Anger, which might relate more properly to misfortune, anger which relates to the client's illness, may sometimes be directed inappropriately as a consequence of projection.

Projection may also involve emotions being attributed to another person. This may be at the root of paranoid ideation, where a person believes that another has hostile feelings towards them. As Stuart and Sundeen (1995, page 573) describe it 'the person who is flooded with unconscious hostile impulses may believe that others are plotting to kill him'. In clinical practice, this may result in difficulties forming relationships with clients or unexpected problems associated with the organization or management of therapeutic interventions. If a client is convinced of the practitioner's hostile intent, attempting to organize a 'social skills programme', for example, is likely to be difficult.

To some extent, projection may be seen even in psychologically healthy individuals. Working relationships are vital to effective community mental health professionals. However, when individuals are faced with difficulties in establishing or maintaining working relationships for reasons which are not immediately apparent, it is worth reflecting as to whether the problem may be the result of projection. The members of a team which is in conflict may find it worth considering whether those involved are really clear as to what the problem is. Could it be related to unconscious feelings which really belong elsewhere? Clients and carers share many qualities; they are both only human. It is vital that the practitioner is aware of the potential impact of projection on both their own behaviour and that of their clients. With this awareness of the potential difficulties involved comes an ability better to understand and deal with otherwise unexplained behaviour and responses.

PSYCHOSOMATIC ILLNESS (*see also* Emotional effects of physical illness; Anxiety management)

This term is often used in a rather perjorative way by some to imply that the illness from which the person is suffering is somehow not quite 'real'. However, illness caused by psychological illness produces the same feelings of ill health as for any illness and thus deserves to be taken seriously. The sufferer may have a variety of physical complaints caused by generalized or specific anxiety, and often feels ashamed of talking about them or conversely, talks about them endlessly, wanting reassurance. Conditions such as ulcers, intestinal disorders, allergies and migraines are seen to be a possible reaction to emotional stress (White and Watt, 1981). The client may be convinced that the illness is purely physical in origin and may not see the links between their symptoms and any underlying emotional links. Medical treatment for their condition can be combined with other measures. For example, the practitioner can offer education about the effects of stress on the body, give emotional support, employ behavioural techniques which may help lessen the effects of the symptoms and encourage the use of relaxation techniques.

QUALITY ASSURANCE (*see also* Standard of care)

Quality assurance programmes and initiatives have developed in response to the Griffiths Report (1983). This report questioned whether the NHS met the needs of its users, and identified that those users include clients, NHS employees, community and the taxpayer. To support the notion of 'quality care' the World Health Organization (1985) recommended that by 1990 effective mechanisms for ensuring quality of client care within the health care systems should be developed.

Quality assurance can be defined as to assure the consumer of a specified degree of excellence through continuous measurement and evaluation (Schmadl, 1979).

Many frameworks have been developed to measure the quality of care in the health care setting. A thorough literature search will enable the choice of a most appropriate model for work area. The first step of the quality cycle is to collaborate with colleagues and develop a philosophy of care. Following this it is necessary to set objectives – what will be achieved by measuring the quality of care. It is necessary to describe what the practitioner does before measuring the quality and to enable this to be done standards and criteria need to be identified (Sale, 1991).

When implementing a quality framework consideration should be given to the elements of a quality service. Maxwell (1984) recommend that accessibility, acceptability, appropriateness, equity, efficiency, and effectiveness are necessary components. In addition, reference to the client group is important. Green (1991) suggests that in mental health care there are additional considerations due to diagnostic difference, the difficulty and the resistance or reluctance of clients to participate in care.

Hostick (1995) suggests that these elements are further complicated by the community setting due to the 'complexity of intervention'. Hostick discusses the development of a quality system within the field of community mental health. The model developed is based upon standard setting and register audit.

The experience of Hostick demonstrated the need for all purchasers to take responsibility for quality measures within their own professional practice and practice area. Effective communication should be maintained with managers to ensure a shared strategy.

R

RATIONAL EMOTIVE THERAPY

Rational emotive therapy was developed by Albert Ellis (1970) as an active-directive cognitively orientated therapy. The underpinning of this therapy is the modification of a person's perceptual set and belief system. Ellis believed that unconscious beliefs lead to maladaptive behaviour. The therapist aids the client to identify their irrational thoughts, re-evaluate the validity of them and through assistance enables the client to discriminate between rational and irrational thinking. Irrational thoughts are reinforced by the negative outcomes that a person predicts, for example if somebody believes that they will fail and says 'I know that I will fail' this creates stress and anxiety leading to tension which in turn eventually leads to failure.

Confrontation is used to force the individual to take responsibility for the behaviour and to accept themselves for what they are rather than what they do. This confrontation along with reality testing corrects the distorted cognitions. The client is taught and encouraged to take new risks and try out new behaviour.

REFERRAL PROCESS (*see also* Appointments)

The way in which a referral will reach the community mental health practitioner will be determined by the team's operational policy. This policy will state whether the referral system is to be 'open' or 'closed'. Open referral systems accept referrals from any source including self-referrals. Closed referral systems limit the source of the referrals. In this system the limitations can vary from team to team but generally the referrals are only accepted from medical personnel such as GPs, consultant psychiatrists and ward doctors. Request for referral can be made verbally by face-to-face contact or by telephone, but it is usually expected that confirmation in writing will follow shortly afterwards. Written referrals are made by letter or by using the team's standard referral form. Other written methods of referral could include sending a copy of the domiciliary visit, outpatient clinic or ward discharge report with a request for follow-up action.

A team has to share its referral policy guidelines with potential referrers and ensure they know how and where to refer, when the service is available, who the team members are, what skills they have to offer and what problems come within their remit.

A referral system has to include a response policy. Depending on whether a referral is routine or urgent, different response times will be involved. The team will need to inform the referrer of receipt of referral and acknowledge its acceptance for allocation. If the referral is inappropriate it will be sent back to the referrer with an explanation or a recommendation to refer to another agency. If a waiting list is in operation, then the referrer and the client should be informed and an estimated waiting time be given. The referrer may be given the opportunity to make a case for prioritizing where there is urgency. Referral allocation will take into account catchment areas, appropriate discipline, team member skills and interests and co-working. A keyworker may be allocated to undertake the initial assessment, or may be appointed after the assessment has been carried out.

The next step in the process is to make the first appointment with the client and inform the referrer of this assessment date.

REFLECTIVE PRACTICE (*see also* Clinical supervision)

The concept of reflective practice is becoming more prevalent in health care practice, particularly nursing, and has become an integral part of any pre-registration or post-registration education. Although much of the literature is focused on education and nursing the concepts of reflective practice can apply to any profession which offers a service to vulnerable others or who are compromised by their role in society.

Reflection in nursing is described by Street (1991) as a way to 'empower nurses to become fully cognisant of their own knowledge, and actions, the person and professional histories which have shaped them, the symbols and images inherent in the language they use, the myths and the metaphors which sustain them in practice, their nursing experiences and the potentialities and constraints of their work setting'.

Put simply, it is examining what you do, how you do it, where you do it, when you do it and why you do it. By questioning the process of a situation

faced in practice, the practitioner is able to take up an opportunity to analyse
the situation and the outcome critically and understand what learning and
professional development has taken place. Although this sounds easy to
achieve, the effects of reflective practice and the importance of the questions
raised cannot be underestimated. 'Reflection is not just thoughtful practice
but a learning experience' (Jarvis, 1992). Reflecting on experience allows practitioners to become more self-aware and self-evaluative.

Methods of reflective practice

There are different ways in which reflective practice can be achieved.

- Reflective frameworks to aid reflection – there are a number of these
  (Johns, 1994; Gibbs, 1988; Goodman, 1984).
- Meeting with other professionals to reflect on practice – this can provide
  support, guidance and allow the opportunity to share and explore with
  another or others.
- Reflective journals or diaries are very useful as they offer a record of
  experiences and reflective process. They are also confidential to the
  writer unless they choose otherwise; often these are used in educational
  courses, and may be used to assist reflection when meeting with other
  professionals.

RELATIONSHIP-BUILDING SKILLS (*see also* Patient or client?)

The ability to establish, develop and maintain a positive and therapeutic
relationship is a skill. This skill is demonstrated when the practitioner is able
to be at ease with people, to put people at ease and to be able to establish a
rapport quickly. During training, existing skills are reflected on, developed
so that they are appropriately used and additional skills are learnt.
Thereafter, relationship-building skills are further developed and refined
through continued professional practice. A relationship is an interaction
between two people. A therapeutic relationship has the mutual intention of
solving a problem. This interaction is the prelude to support, assessment
and therapy. Some interventions can be carried out without the benefit of a
relationship and some degree of assessment can be undertaken, but this
would entail the assessor's observations alone. The assessment would lack
the client's perception of the problem and their involvement in the treatment plan. The intervention would be prescriptive; a relationship assumes a
partnership and with this latter approach, the passive patient expecting a
cure becomes the client involved in the decision-making and problem-
solving processes. When developing a relationship, at the first meeting the
community practitioner uses the skills identified by various counsellors and
therapists, but in particular the ideas explored in writings of Carl Rogers

(1951; 1961). The practitioner creates what is sometimes called a 'therapeutic milieu'. An atmosphere of trust is facilitated by the practitioner's expression of empathy, warmth and genuineness.

Empathy

The skilled practitioner has the ability accurately to perceive and reflect back both the affective and cognitive experiences of the client. When this happens successfully, the client feels that the practitioner understands or at least is trying very hard to understand.

Unconditional positive regard

A term first used by Carl Rogers. This involves, on the part of the practitioner, an attitude of respect for the client as a person. This attitude displays in the form of acceptance regardless of the individual's behaviour, and necessitates the avoidance of any judgement by the practitioner.

Genuineness

This refers to the practitioner's ability to be authentic. The client feels that the practitioner is genuinely interested and not assuming the role of counsellor. The non-verbal expression of warmth and concern also serve to reassure the client of the practitioner's genuineness. The relationship is further developed by the presentation of listening and attending skills. Clients value the opportunity to offload, to get concerns off their chest, to put words to how they feel and to release bottled-up feelings of frustration, anger and anxiety. Often, all they ask for is 'a person who is prepared to listen'. The practitioner's responding skills enable the relationship to move forward and tentative exploration of the problem areas takes place (Egan, 1982), for example 'I wonder if ...'; 'could it be that ...'; 'what have you tried so far ...'. At this stage relationship formation has taken place. The client feels safe to confide and now has a safe base from which to work. The client has confidence in the practitioner's competence, skills and experience; the practitioner has been 'assessed' by the client.

RELAXATION TECHNIQUES (*see also* Anxiety management; Alerts and emergencies)

Day centres often run groups specifically for the purpose of teaching relaxation techniques. However, it may be appropriate to teach individual clients these techniques so that they can use them in their own homes when it is most convenient to them. They can be used to relieve the symptoms of stress and anxiety such as fatigue, aches and pains and tension.

Different techniques can be employed by the client depending on the strength of their feelings. For example, a first step may be that the client recognizes the difference between tension and relaxation by using a set of progressive movements that contrasts the two states. The anxious or stressed person may be so used to the state of continually tensed muscles that they will find the contrast quite difficult to make at first. Encouraging them to accompany this practice with deep breathing or some music that they find soothing will help. A relaxation technique can also be taught for use in times of extreme panic or distress. The client is asked to sit down and say 'stop' sharply to themselves, following this with a deep breath. On breathing out slowly, the shoulders should be allowed to drop. After inhaling again, this time while exhaling, concentration should focus on dropping the jaw and chin towards the neck. This cycle can be repeated for a few minutes. For the client who wants to use relaxation techniques regularly at home, it may be useful to provide them with a cassette tape which has pre-recorded instructions. There are many of these available on the market, but it might be valuable to record a personal one as the client is familiar with the sound of the practitioner's voice and may be able to identify more easily with this.

Teaching massage may be another technique that the client can use at home with family or friends. This has the added benefit of reducing the isolation that is often felt by those suffering from anxiety and tension. A non-threatening form of massage should be taught on the hands, face, neck or shoulders, using a perfumed or non-perfumed oil, and the client should be encouraged to feed back their feelings both during and after the massage.

REMINISCENCE THERAPY AND REALITY ORIENTATION

The onset of confusion, disorientation and memory loss relating to the development of irreversible mental illness causes anxiety and concern amongst clients and families alike wherever it occurs. Care in the community presents particular challenges for the management of individuals who are experiencing confusion and disorientation. Too often, despair and hopelessness or, perhaps even more disturbingly, resigned acceptance meet the onset of organic mental illness in the community. Reality orientation and reminiscence therapy approaches are active ways to approach the management of such clients, based as they are on an assumption that the person with mental health problems has the same right to information and guidance as any other person in our society. Reality orientation is best considered as a philosophy or an approach to care which incorporates a feeling and an understanding that there is value in talking to elderly, confused people and that by using varying approaches to meet the multiple deficits and abilities of these individuals, communication and cognitive deficits can be alleviated.

A number of approaches need to be taken by the therapist working in a community setting when dealing with confused clients. One key area involves the use of relatives, friends and significant others in assisting the client to new levels of orientation through their day-to-day interactions, the so-called '24-hour reality orientation approach'. It is important to point out to visitors and carers the importance to the client of a consistent, accurate approach, confirming reality, rather than simply agreeing with the client's inaccurate perceptions. Clearly, support for carers is a vital part of this process for the community practitioner (Kempton, 1984).

A development of the reality orientation approach involves providing cues to the client to reinforce such cognitive functioning as remains. Myles (1991) considers the use of such subtle approaches to be vital. In the client's home, this could involve the use of prompts and signs which may assist the client in finding their way about and maximizing their independent functioning. Sometimes criticized as 'institutionalizing' a house, this is clearly worthwhile if it assists the client in their orientation.

Reminiscence constitutes an important part of day-to-day interaction with the confused client. Looking back over more distant memories, and linking them to the issues of today, may assist the disorientated client in coping more effectively with the issues to be faced in daily life in their own home.

Reality orientation and reminiscence together may make a considerable difference to the confused client. It also provides an important task and approach for those who care for them, providing a meaningful and considered approach to helping their relative more effectively.

RESOURCE CENTRES

Resource centres are multidisciplinary community centres set up and functioning within the community setting. Obviously each centre has its own operational policy but in the main the following occur.

- **Walk in service** – anyone can walk in and be seen by a health professional for assessment of their mental health needs.
- **Multidisciplinary collaborative working** – all professionals function as keyworkers and carry caseloads.
- **Therapeutic programme** – centres run a therapeutic programme involving group work, individual counselling and therapies including art, music and so on. These programmes are accessed on a sessional basis, but clients may attend for one or two days if necessary.

This is a very broad overview of the resource centre model and in some aspects it duplicates the day hospital model except it is totally separate from the hospital environment. Often community mental health practitioners are based at resource centres and use the facilities to see clients as well as visiting clients at home. It may be argued that this type of centre reduces the stigma of mental illness by bringing it to the community; a further advantage is its accessibility which may help clients to seek help before crisis occurs.

S

SCHIZOPHRENIA (*see also* Delusions; Hallucinations)

Schizophrenia is characterized by severe disturbance of thinking, feelings and behaviour. There is increasing social withdrawal and the sufferer is usually pre-occupied with delusional beliefs and hallucinations. The illness is often chronic with periods of remission or acute exacerbation. This century there has been a dramatic shift in the care of the person with schizophrenia, progressing from custodial care to community care. This has been via the approaches of physical–medical treatments and social psychiatry. In the community, medical treatments are made available thereby reducing the need for hospital admissions. When admissions are necessary, the periods of stay have become increasingly shorter, instigated at an earlier stage of a relapse and involve more continuity of care between the community and the hospital. Shorter stays in hospital have resulted in far less risk of clients becoming institutionalized and developing the secondary condition described by Barton (1959) in which clients display an apathy and passivity that is not part of the primary psychotic illness. An important medical treatment for schizophrenia is the use of antipsychotic drugs that can alleviate an acute phase of the illness or maintain progress by reducing the likelihood or severity of future episodes. Drug treatment is not a cure for schizophrenia but does reduce some of the distressing symptoms and make clients more amenable to the psychological and social approaches used by mental health practitioners. These major tranquillizers can be administered orally or in the form of long-acting depot injections.

Community care has increased the opportunities for social treatments, enabling the community mental health practitioners to take into account environmental, leisure, family, work and accommodation factors. These social factors may be a source of stress for clients and, conversely, a source of support. Much of the skill in treating schizophrenia is in arranging an environment that is optimally stimulating. With insufficient stimulation negative symptoms increase; with too much stimulation positive symptoms become more pronounced (Gelder *et al.*, 1994). The positive symptoms of schizophrenia could be described as abnormal psychological factors such as delusions, hallucinations and thought disorders, and the negative symptoms as diminished or absent normal functions such as poverty of speech, flattening of affect, loss of volition, withdrawal and apathy (Fottrell, 1983). For clients to function at their optimal level, a balance of the social factors is striven for. For practitioners to be in a position to help clients, trusting relationships need to be established. When clients have schizophrenia, the building of relationships can present a difficult task for practitioners. Clients' expressions of their delusional beliefs, their alternative perception of reality, language disorders and incongruent affect can be a challenge to the practitioner's attempts to empathize. If clients perceive a lack of empathy and feel misunderstood, then hostility and suspicion can result. It has sometimes been said that there is a 'glass wall' between us and a schizophrenic. It may seem like this viewed from the non-psychotic side of the barrier. From his side there is no wall (Crowcroft, 1967). Practitioners may have difficulty perceiving clients' attitudes to intervention due to this 'glass wall' but clients will soon perceive a practitioner's anxiety and lack of interest or genuineness. Many of the conventional communication skills taught may not be applicable in relationships with schizophrenics who may feel threatened by physical closeness, touch, eye contact and attempts to talk (Brooking *et al.*, 1992). The benefits of 'talking treatments', that is counselling and psychotherapy, have been questioned by some authors, while others feel that as long as the therapy is 'supportive' and 'resocializing' rather than 'dynamic' or 'analytical' then over-stimulation and defensiveness on the part of clients may be avoided.

Once a rapport has been established and practitioners have regular contact with clients, then care plan goals can be considered. When working with such a complex illness as schizophrenia, practitioners will need to work closely with the families of clients and with colleagues within the multi-disciplinary team. Medication and mental health monitoring will need to be shared with the doctor responsible for the client. Liaison with a social worker or care manager will take place when there are issues around accommodation, finance or self-neglect and more practical help is required. For clients living alone, occupational therapy assessment and involvement can be useful in enabling them to develop the skills of daily living needed to cope more independently. Psychologists can undertake assessment and advise on or treat behaviour difficulties. The short-term goals of a care plan may focus on the basic and practical day-to-day issues of nutritional needs, safety, warmth, accommodation, social support network and compliance with medication. The longer term goals may be to assist clients in under-standing and coping with their illness, to maintain their optimal level of independence, and retain the care and support of their family and friends. The practitioner's support of formal and informal carers is important when clients are faced with a life event, as the associated stress can increase the chance of positive or negative symptoms appearing. Where there is emotional over-involvement between clients and their families, practitioners may be able to arrange day care or respite for the client to reduce this contact and thereby lessen the risk of relapse. The family of a person with schizophrenia can suffer social embarrassment, depression, anxiety, fear and guilt. Practitioners may find that time spent counselling carers can be time well spent, as a family that is supported is more likely to be able to continue caring. It is also worth putting carers in touch with voluntary organizations including The National Schizophrenic Fellowship, MIND (National Association for Mental Health), and The Richmond Fellowship, so that further information, advice and support can be given.

SELF-HELP GROUPS

Self-help groups are generally developed and organized by the membership of the group, but the community mental health practitioner is in an excellent position to get together clients with similar needs and problems. It is important that confidentiality be maintained and permission sought when talking to clients about setting up a group. In the main the members operate the group themselves without a professional group facilitator or leader. The aim of the group is to solve problems raised by the members, to share their concerns, anxieties and to gain support and understanding from others with whom they can identify. Although famous self-help groups such as Alcoholics Anonymous and Gamblers Anonymous are known for focus-ing on repressing and abstaining from impulses, many of the groups focus on sharing feelings about an illness and the recognition of not being alone with one's symptoms.

To work effectively in the community the practitioner should be aware of all self-help groups, the aims and focus of the groups and a contact number or name. If the practitioner should feel that a self-help group is appropriate for a group of clients, then after checking that none suitable is already avail-able, he or she should suggest to each of them the opportunity of talking to another about their illness. *Permission from each client should be sought* before introducing them to each other. *Confidentiality* should be main-tained and the clients should be enabled to set up the group themselves.

Obviously the practitioner can assist with resources and accommodation as much as possible, but it is up to the clients to identify their ground rules, the focus of the group and so on. The practitioner who attends a group will gain valuable insight into the strength and impact of self-help groups.

SETTING UP SUPERVISION (*see also* Clinical supervision; Management supervision)

Although there is much literature on clinical supervision, there is little published on how to set up clinical supervision within one's work area. This section seeks to offer a guide to this.

Clinical supervision may occur on a one to one, group or peer basis. The first job is to find a supervisor that a practitioner feels confident of. It is imperative that this person be able to challenge, support and enable them to empower themselves to develop. The other person must, of course, be willing to supervise. It may be tempting to choose a friend or colleague to whom the practitioner relates well; although this is fine, they must ensure that their supervisor will be objective and not collude with them.

Training for both supervisor and supervisee roles is recommended (Butterworth, 1994; Kohner, 1994) but obviously not always available. It is therefore necessary to try to examine literature relating to clinical supervision and grasp a fuller understanding.

The following is necessary when forming a supervision relationship.

1. Set ground rules, time, place, cancellation policy, regularity, note keeping, confidentiality rules and so on. It may be that the practitioner's organization has a policy, procedure and standard for clinical supervision in place. Unless the organization has identified frequency of meetings and length of time of meetings there are no strict guidelines.
2. Ensure that both supervisee and supervisor have a full understanding of the type of supervision expected. If a structure model is to be used (e.g. Proctor, 1986) then this should be identified.
3. Set evaluation dates, to offer the choice for both parties to examine the progress of the supervision.

Guidance for supervisee

1. Use your time effectively, after all it is *your* time.
2. If you have difficulty identifying an issue to discuss, then perhaps you are looking *too* hard, or for complications which do not exist.
3. At first you may feel frustrated that your supervisor does not produce answers to your concerns; recognize that she is seeking to enable you to find the answers through developing yourself and therefore your practice.
4. At first it may feel difficult to talk to another person about your practice. Give it time and soon you will look forward to supervision and wonder how you managed so long without it.

5. Keep your own records: these may be open or closed and should be retained to enable you to examine your own development (by looking back over your notes). These also act as a reminder when recapping in the next session.

Guidance for supervisor

1. There may be temptation at first to 'sort out the problem' or issue for the supervisee. Remember that your role is to enable the supervisee to sort out their issues not you.
2. Remain objective, however difficult this is.
3. Always negotiate in ground rules that if malpractice has occurred then in the first instance you will allow the supervisee to inform their manager but if this does not occur you will have to take the issue further and report it (UKCC, 1984a).
4. Keep records for monitoring and audit purposes.
5. Give guidance when necessary.
6. Supervision is *not* a conversation.
7. There is a need for the supervisor to be up to date on current nursing issues and policies and to be coherent with all UKCC guidelines.

Issues regarding the supervisor

A hierarchical profession like nursing encourages hierarchical approaches to clinical supervision and in many areas choice has not been offered to the supervisee. Advantages and disadvantages regarding having a manager as supervisor are listed by Kohner (1994). In mental health care a multidisciplinary approach already exists and is developing further; this may entail different professions supervising each other. This is acceptable when focused primarily on clinical aspects of care, but clinical supervision for nurses entails a professional nursing aspect. Identification of the aims and objectives of multidisciplinary supervision is required and if this occurs regularly and often then clinical supervision (nursing) could be reduced.

SEXUALITY (*see also* Sexual problems)

This is an area sometimes not given enough importance by practitioners, possibly because of the social taboos that surround the subject, the fear of offending the client, or even the embarrassment of the practitioner who may feel uncomfortable about discussing such a personal issue. However, sexuality, or the picture one has of oneself, is at the core of the client's existence and is often threatened at times of mental or emotional crisis.

Kucynski (1980) argues that sexuality is a complex area, encompassing not only behaviour linked to sexual activity but also to one's self concept and identity – the way one expresses feelings and beliefs about oneself.

Illness of any type may alter clients' perception of themselves. For example, during a depressive illness, or after surgery, the client may feel a loss of sexual identity and it is therefore important to explore this sensitively. The practitioner could ask questions such as 'has your illness affected the way you feel about yourself?' or 'can you tell me how you feel about yourself at the moment?'. These questions may encourage clients to talk about an area that may be very important to them, but that until now they have felt should be kept hidden. Illness or medication may have also caused direct effects on their sexual behaviour which the client finds distressing and explanations will offer some reassurance.

Cultural expectations of sexuality may lead to stereotyping or judgemental attitudes, however careful the practitioner is, and this can affect the therapeutic relationship from both sides. Clients, for example, may find expressing personal ideas about themselves to someone of the opposite sex difficult, or practitioners may make assumptions about specific behaviour expected from male or female clients. Gender may also affect the way in which symptoms are presented or discussed.

SEXUAL PROBLEMS (*see also* Sexuality)

Sexual problems are common for those suffering any type of emotional or mental health problems. Many of the drugs prescribed in themselves have a physical effect on the client. Phenothiazines such as chlorpromazine may reduce sexual interest and cause retarded or absent ejaculation, as is also the case with tricyclic anti-depressants, MAOIs and lithium carbonate (Hawton, 1985). Depression is a particularly common precipitant, causing loss of interest and often a complete cessation of intercourse after the start of the depressive symptoms. Stress and anxiety can also have an effect, not just on the sexual life of clients but also on how clients feel about their general body image and sexuality. However, clients may feel embarrassed to confess to these feelings and may not always link them to their ill health problems or to the medication that they have been prescribed. The effect of these sexual problems may add to the consequences of the client's illness on their existing relationships, particularly if there is a lack of communication and understanding. It is understandable that both clients and practitioners may be hesitant about discussing sexual problems, yet the practitioner should take the lead in initiating helpful interventions. For example, it may be useful to ask a general question such as 'how has your illness affected your life with your husband/wife/ partner?', or 'are there any worries that you have about the effects of your medication or treatment on your sex life?'. A gentle approach into a sensitive area may provide the client with the opportunity needed to ventilate their feelings. The practitioner can offer then to discuss this with the client, particularly in order to provide reassurance that what is being experienced is not abnormal, but is a natural consequence of their condition or medication. The practitioner's role here is of information giver and offerer of support through their changed picture of themselves. This may extend to the client's partner in order to give the practitioner further opportunities to reassure and explain what is happening. However, there may be occasions when the conditions experienced are either causing severe disruption to normal life or have existed for longer than could be expected. In these cases, unless the practitioner is skilled in psychosexual counselling, referral should be made to a specialist counsellor or service such as Relate.

SIDE EFFECTS OF MEDICATION (*see also* Medication and mental health)

The majority of neuroleptic drugs carry side effects ranging from mild to severe. *The British National Formulary* (BMA, 1996) is an invaluable aid for the practitioner, and it is a recommended book to be available at all times, giving detailed accounts of all groups of medication that are prescribed and the side effects that can be expected. The client who has been prescribed a new or different medication should also be educated about side effects, not in order to frighten them but so that they will recognize symptoms for what they are and be able to report them to either the practitioner or the GP so that help can be given quickly. The main side effects of different drug groups are as follows but this is not an exhaustive list such as can be found in the *Formulary*.

- **Benzodiazepine drugs** such as diazepam, which are prescribed for the short-term relief of anxiety, can cause drowsiness or unsteadiness, enough to affect one's ability to drive or coordinate properly. The elderly are particularly sensitive and the drug can cause confusion. Regular monitoring is advised for those taking such drugs over a long period and withdrawal should be gradual.
- **Anti-psychotic drugs** such as chlorpromazine have a wide range of side effects, including extrapyramidal symptoms such as tremor, restlessness, hypotension and pronounced sedative effects. Clients taking these types of drugs should also be advised that the skin becomes hypersensitive to the sun and a sunblock should be used at all times during hot weather.
- **Lithium carbonate**, used in the treatment of manic depressive illness, can also result in a variety of side effects including gastro-intestinal upsets, tremor and muscle weakness. Three monthly checks should be done for lithium levels in the blood, and severe overdosage can cause convulsions,

toxic psychosis and circulatory failure. Finally antidepressants such as amitriptyline can cause dry mouth, blurred vision, constipation and urinary retention.

It is apparent from this brief overview that a detailed knowledge of side effects benefits both the practitioner and the client. Some of the side effects can be distressing to the client and yet can be easily remedied once noticed.

SOCIAL SKILLS TRAINING

Social skills training has been used extensively within the area of mental health care. In the main it is used to enable those who lack social skills, for instance some clients who have experienced long-term institutionalization and for those who are phobic of social situations. More often than not clients will present with both these difficulties.

Group training is most effective and sessions may be for up to two hours for a specific period, for instance 10–12 weeks. Group size should be no more than ten if possible. Group facilitators consist of one person to take overall responsibility for running the group along with two co-facilitators.

Prior to referral to the group, the client is assessed and identified goals or targets will be formulated with the individual. Measurements of anxiety, depression and current social skills functioning will be made.

The sessions will involve role-plays of specific social situations. These may be video-taped which will allow for feedback on performance. Both strengths and weaknesses of performance will be highlighted and alternatives designed to change behaviour and develop skills will be suggested. Only feedback on the observable behaviour demonstrated is discussed. The group facilitator may demonstrate or 'model' the appropriate behaviour first, then request that the client repeat the role play. Coaching and prompting will be given until the performance is satisfactory. Follow-up work or homework is given at the end of each session and the clients are encouraged to maintain a diary of their relevant social interactions. This is fed back at the start of each session.

Prior to commencing a group it is important for inexperienced practitioners to join as co-facilitator and undertake further study of available literature.

STANDARD OF CARE (*see also* Quality assurance)

Defining standards provides a clear definition of an agreed level of performance for practitioners. It is a measure against which current practice can be compared.

To set standards requires the following:

1. a framework to ensure that all components are considered;
2. consideration of who is the right person to set the standards.

Standard setting frameworks are plentiful and include Donabedian (1980), Crosby (1989), and Maxwell (1984). For the purposes of this section, the Donabedian model of structure, process and outcome will be used. The Donabedian framework has been used extensively in nursing (Kitson, 1985; Kitson, 1988; Kendall, 1988).

Writing the standard statement

This involves defining the 'standard statement' and describing the objective of the standard. It is suggested that the following be considered:

- the standard statement should have a clearly defined target group at which the standard is aimed;
- which individual or group of individuals is responsible for maintaining the standard;
- be within the sphere of influence of those setting the standard;
- should be a clear statement of intent.

In addition standard statements should be SMART: Specific, Measurable, Achievable, Relevant and Theoretically based. Three different criteria are described by Donabedian (1980) as necessary to meet the standard:

1. **structure criteria** – resources required to meet the standard;
2. **process criteria** – actions required by individuals in order to meet the standard;
3. **outcome criteria** – the desired effect of the standard in terms of behaviour.

This piece is merely an overview on standard setting and the author recommends that prior to setting standards within a practice area, further reading and a literature search is made.

STRESS AND COPING (*see also* Reflective practice; Clinical supervision)

The stressful nature of nursing was identified by Menzies (1960). Although this study focused on the general nurse the stressors identified were relevant to all nurses. In particular the stressful effect of the emotionally demanding nature of relationships was explored. This, combined with the findings of Holsclaw (1965) that working with patients with psychiatric problems and being unable to restore patients to well-being was an emotionally high risk area, raises the expectation that mental health nursing is indeed stressful. Despite these findings very few studies of stress in psychiatric nursing have been performed. It appears that only one study (Carson *et al.*, 1995) has focused upon stress and the community psychiatric nurse.

A pioneer in the study of stress Hans Selye defines stress purely in physiological terms as 'non specific response of the body to the demands made upon it' (Selye, 1956). He described his model of stress as the General Adaptation Syndrome and included three stages:

1. **the alarm reaction** – when the individual becomes aware of the situation and the stressors;
2. **the resistant stage** – this is when the homeostatic mechanisms of the body are mobilized to adjust to the stressor;
3. **the exhaustion stage** – this is if homeostasis is not restored and stress persists causing eventual morbidity.

Stressors

Lazarus (1971) identified that stress could be described as internal or external to the individual. Internal stressors can be described as personal ambition, high standards that an individual sets for themselves and so on. External stressors may include relationship difficulties, job demands, loss of job or change of role. In 1978 Lazarus and Launier highlighted the important effects of psychological stress which could enable the enhancement of performance but showed that if the demands exceeded the resources required then negative physical and psychological responses may occur. An individual's perception of a stressor may determine the response and Lazarus (1970) developed this further by postulating that stress reactions are directly related to the cognitive appraisal of the situation by the individual.

Difficulties occur when the demands of a stressor exceed the resources of the individual's coping system. Coping with stress commences when the equilibrium between demands and resources is disturbed. Lazarus and Launier (1978) identified four modes of coping. These are:

- the search for information
- direct action
- inhibition of action
- intro-psychic defence.

A combination of these methods may be used and it is solely dependent upon the situation.

Burnout

Burnout was described by Freudenberger (1974) as 'a syndrome of physical and emotional exhaustion experienced by those in the helping professions when they feel overwhelmed by other people's problems'. Maslac (1979) and Cherniss (1980) have identified that the sufferer develops a negative job attitude, loss of concern and feelings for clients and experiences changes in motivation which include loss of enthusiasm and purpose at work. Three general stages of burnout have been identified by Spaniel and Capputo (1978), Maslac (1979) and Prophit (personal communication, 1983). These are as follows.

1. Symptoms are experienced occasionally, but the individual feels emotionally and physically exhausted.
2. Symptoms become more regular and last longer and cynical dehumanizing attitudes towards clients develop. At this stage the individual may become withdrawn.
3. The symptoms become chronic, the individual questions his or her work and is unable to control emotions; there may be manifestations of other physical symptoms.

Identifying and being aware of stressors is the first step toward coping successfully and preventing the negative effects of stress and finally burnout.

STRESSORS AND COMMUNITY MENTAL HEALTH CARE

Appleby (1992) has suggested that the sources of stress in mental health care can be divided into four broad areas:

1. factors relating to psychiatric nursing care;
2. the individual factors in nurses;
3. organizational factors;
4. factors relating to changes in psychiatric nursing.

So what are the stressors of being a community mental health nurse? McCallion (1989) performed a survey of 25 rural community psychiatric nurses to identify the main stressors of their professional role. At that time the CPNs identified that their main stressors were: dogs, isolation, lack of support, concern over future role and lack of control over future of the service. An examination of whether burnout was present highlighted that a number of the nurses used negative coping strategies. These were smoking, increased alcohol intake and increased food intake. Carson *et al.* (1995) surveyed 250 CPNs to identify the top ten stressors for a community psychiatric nurse. They are as follows.

1. Not having facilities in the community to which clients can be referred.
2. Knowing there are long waiting lists before clients can get access to services.

3. Having to deal with suicidal clients alone.
4. Not having enough time to study or personal improvement.
5. Trying to keep up a good quality of care in work.
6. Having too many interruptions when trying to work in the office.
7. Having to visit unsafe areas.
8. Feeling there is not enough hospital backup.
9. Having to work with clients with a known history of violence.
10. Having to cope with changes at the work place.

Carson *et al.* also identified that CPNs who scored low on the CPN stress questionnaire took on average 4.8 days off sick in the past year. For the high stress group the number of sickness days was 11.1. The authors recommend that stress reducing interventions can provide a variety of levels and suggest four different ways this may occur.

1. Individual CPNs who have problems coping be offered individual stress management.
2. Groups of CPNs within a district service be offered a group based approach tethered to their local circumstances.
3. Health providers be encouraged to offer stress reduction packages for all staff of which CPNs constitute only a small part.
4. It might be helpful to monitor the effects of wider scale service changes on CPNs.

Nurses are afraid of being seen as unstable, weak or incompetent and expressing negative emotions (Mulling and Barstow, 1979). Jones (1982) suggests that nurses are socialized in believing that it is unacceptable for a good nurse to admit feelings of stress. Methods of preventing and reducing stress and burnout include educational interventions such as stress management courses, assertiveness training and developing self-awareness skills. Reflection on practice is a way of turning experience into learning and writing about personal experiences: it can aid the exploration of emotions and anxieties and help the nurse to recognize particular stressors. It is commonplace now for a student nurse to keep a diary whilst in the clinical area to enable their self-development process as well as proving a record of significant learning experiences (Walker, 1985). *Ad hoc* peer support at work has always been a way of reducing and preventing stress. This stems from colleagues being sensitive to each other's needs and from meetings of informal or formal support groups on a regular basis. Clinical supervision should be available to all nurses to enable the exploration of the effect of stress and stressors in relation to their nursing practice. Additionally time management courses are particularly appropriate for all community nurses so that they are not rushing from client to client creating more tension and more stress, not worrying about getting caught up in traffic jams and making sure that there is time in between visits for themselves. This allows recharge of batteries and enables practitioners to give the most to each client that they see.

There is a need for community mental health nurses to recognize the effects of stress and the sources of stress within their working role. It is imperative that they can be assertive, manage their time effectively and feel valued about the work which they perform. It is important that they move away from feeling guilty when stressed and from thinking that they are 'not a good nurse' if they experience stress. Stress can be an enhancer: it can help people work more effectively, it can enable someone to achieve, but for this to occur, the resources have to be available within the individual to work under that level of pressure for a long period of time.

STUDENTS

Community mental health teams provide excellent learning environments for students from a variety of disciplines. While they are popular placements for the students, having students does pose certain problems which do not occur in institutional settings where students can fairly easily be absorbed into the routine of the ward. A student who has not had any prior experience of community working may well feel apprehensive and vulnerable at first, finding it hard to see how they can fit in. This should be appreciated and alleviated by the team identifying the practitioner with whom the student will be linked for the majority of the time, who can then be responsible for introducing the other members of the team and their various functions. Strong links between the placement and the college or training establishment will also enable the student to have a clear idea of the type of team to which they are going in advance. If students have not been given a set of learning objectives to be achieved during their placement, then the responsible practitioner should work with the student on identifying realistic goals that can be achieved during the placement. As soon as possible after starting work with the team, it is useful for the student to go out in order to get to know the area in which they will be placed and the factors such as culture, economics and employment which influence the lives of clients. The motivation level of students coming to work in the community is generally high and there is usually a feeling of wanting to 'get going' which can lead to frustration unless the student understands quickly the nature of community work and the needs of clients, which can mean that it will not always be appropriate for the student to accompany the practitioner on all home visits. Once students are aware of this and accept that it is not a personal slight, they are usually quite happy to arrange alternative activities for the times when the practitioner is busy with existing clients. This also means that they undertake as wide a range of community experiences as possible, such as visits to day centres, rehabilitation units, addiction teams and so on.

Students who are inexperienced or on short placements obviously will not take on clients of their own, but will, by watching the practitioner at work, gain an understanding of the extent of therapeutic interventions that are possible in the community. Students who are on longer placements will be able, with supervision, to take on a small caseload that is congruent with their experience and skills. This is obviously something that needs a good knowledge of the student and an awareness of the client's needs. Working closely with the whole team ensures that the student does not feel unsupported and that there is always someone to hand for discussion of the progress that is being made. Similarly, referrals to the student should be made only after team discussion with the student present. The practitioner may decide to accompany the student on at least the first visit, and thereafter until the student feels confident to continue alone. Even then, the practitioner, being still the accountable person, must insist on records being kept in the same format as the rest of the team and on all clinical procedures being observed. The dilemma frequently expressed by practitioners is of 'letting go' of the student, and this can only be comfortably settled by thorough observation of, and discussion with, the student and the rest of the team since although a student may appear highly confident, the practitioner is always aware of the vulnerability of the client and the potential damage that could be done by a student who is not ready to work on a one to one basis.

SUPERVISION REGISTER

Supervision registers were introduced by the Department of Health in April 1994. Their introduction was announced in December 1993 as a response to a series of highly publicized incidents involving people with mental illnesses: these included Ben Silcott climbing into a lion's cage at London Zoo and the killing of Jonathan Zito by Christopher Clunis.

Guidance on the requirements of supervision registers is contained in HSG(94)5 issued by the NHS Management Executive on 10 February 1994 (DOH, 1994 b). The purpose of supervision registers is to: 'Identify all individuals who are under the care of an NHS Provider Unit known to be at significant risk of committing serious violence or suicide or of serious self neglect as a result of severe and enduring mental illness'. For the purpose of the supervision registers psychopathic disorders are included as serious and enduring mental illnesses.

The responsibility for placing a client on a supervision register rests with the consultant psychiatrist but the guidance recommends that the decision is made through consultation with the multidisciplinary team. The guidance also recommends that the patient is informed of the decision to place them on the register except where it is thought that such information may damage their health. It is likely, in most cases, that the keyworker appointed for a client on the supervision register will be a CPN. Before seeing the client for the first time after they have been placed on the register it is essential to know the reason for registration and what discussion there has been with the client about the decision. By definition these clients are the most at risk and/or pose the greatest risk to others; as such, clarity and consistency of communication is even more critical to establishing a therapeutic relationship.

T

TERMINATING A RELATIONSHIP (*see also* Standard of care)

The aims of working in the community with clients can vary widely. Some clients may never regain totally independent functioning, and the practitioner, as part of the multidisciplinary team may be involved in long-term support and monitoring of their condition. Others, after brief interventions, are able to move back to an autonomous life style. However, both time restrictions and size of caseload on the part of the practitioner and the danger of dependency on the practitioner by the client mean that the duration of the relationship needs to be considered carefully. When working with clients whose needs appear to require short-term help, the practitioner can, from the start of the relationship, explain the extent of the help which can be offered and the expected length of time that will need to be spent working on the presenting problems. This gives the client an idea of the boundaries of the relationship and does not give false expectations that the practitioner will always be around. It can also be explained that this is negotiable and will depend on frequent review of the progress that the client is making.

TRANSCULTURAL ISSUES IN MENTAL HEALTH CARE

Major difficulties exist in mental health services to black and ethnic minority groups. The principal cause of this and its effects were identified as:

- less likelihood of alternatives to hospital admission being offered;
- restrictions to psychotherapy and counselling;
- higher incidence of admission and UK mental heath legislation;

- more likely to be diagnosed as suffering from schizophrenia or psychotic illness;
- detained in 'locked' wards;
- regarded as 'dangerous' and treated accordingly (DoH, 1993b; MIND, 1993).

There is a failure to recognize and accept concepts of mental health from other cultures or to take account of the effects of racism and socio-economic factors. The community mental health practitioner is at the forefront of enabling changes to occur within services to ethnic minority groups. Racism of all forms must be identified, recognized and its problems solved. To offer an improved service practitioners need to consider the following areas:

1. equal opportunity to services for all clients;
2. adequate appropriate and accessible service provision which meets the needs of all sections of the community;
3. the development of services for all groups;
4. the offer of an interpreter or translator as necessary and to ensure understanding of function and working of services;
5. ensuring that thorough information is given (by interpreter if necessary) about medication, illness and treatment;
6. identification of service deficits in relation to ethnic groups.

It is therefore recommended that nurses examine ethnic records and monitoring data in order to evaluate services available fully. This includes gaining access to information which focuses on:

- **access** – who is receiving services and by what process;
- **quality** – appropriateness: what types of service are being provided and do they meet the needs of all ethnic groups in the local population?
- **adequacy** – are services adequate to meet the needs of all ethnic groups in the local population; using this information for evaluation, local practice can develop.

Communication can be more effective by using simple methods:

- all important information should be provided in English and most commonly used languages;
- leaflets on important health issues including The Mental Health Act should be available in English and most commonly used languages;
- leaflets and posters should reflect the multiracial makeup of the population including white.

In the community there may be local and voluntary groups which have been created to meet the needs of the multiracial component of the local population. The community mental health practitioner should seek out, liaise with and gain advice and help from these groups as appropriate to ensure a comprehensive access to service.

TRANSFERENCE AND COUNTER-TRANSFERENCE (*see also* Clinical supervision)

Amongst the many hazards which a mental health worker has to face in the community, transference and counter-transference may be amongst the most potent. As ego or mental defence mechanisms, they are linked back to ideas of psychoanalytical concepts of the self. The experiences of one's past, and especially of childhood, continue to have an influence even though no longer consciously recognized: they have an impact on the way in which personality and values develop and on the ability of the individual to cope with psychological stress.

Transference occurs when a person, most often a client, begins to focus onto the therapist or practitioner the emotions which properly should belong to another person, most often seen as a parent. The emotion is commonly associated with love and affection, but can equally be negative and hostile or distrustful. The consequence of this may be a particular hazard to the person working in the community, because the relative isolation from other staff members may make it less likely that it will be recognized by other colleagues, and subsequently dealt with.

At times, transference may be confused with genuine liking, or even sexual attraction. This poses particular dangers to the practitioner who may find themselves responding inappropriately to the client quite unconsciously. This unconscious response is known as counter-transference, and has precisely the same origins. Transference and counter-transference (from the therapist to the client) occur unconsciously. There needs to be an awareness of the dangers to the therapeutic relationship of these insidious and damaging processes. Transference may be used by the practitioner in a variety of ways. It may assist the client to achieve goals which would otherwise not be possible and may therefore sometimes be helpful. It can provide a focus for moving the therapeutic relationship on beyond the point it would otherwise reach.

Clinical supervision of practice should assist in avoiding this process, but it is still a potential problem for all community practitioners. Individuals finding themselves faced with developing emotional relationships within their work with clients in the community need to consider their professional relationship further. Sharing feelings with a colleague, a manager or a supervisor is required. The feelings are not something one can prevent, but they need to be understood and managed to ensure that the client is not hurt and professional relationships are maintained.

WOMEN AND MENTAL HEALTH

In mental illness statistics, women are over represented. The RCN document *Health of Half the Nation* (RCN, 1992) depicts a gloomy picture: high levels of psychotropic medication prescriptions, increased admission to acute psychiatric inpatient care, diagnoses of depression, illness and Alzheimer's disease and little access to alternative therapies.

The rationale for these figures includes women's place within society as that of the oppressed, along with predominantly male doctors. Enhanced levels of stress (MIND, 1992) from birth to old age are encountered along with expected patterns of behaviour. Additionally abuse, whether sexual, verbal or physical, may be encountered. Women's specific roles like those of motherhood and carer, not only exacerbate distress but catalyse it to create a disequilibrium of mental health. It is suggested that contact with mental health services may cause further distress.

Although evidence suggests that social, economic and political factors create more vulnerability of women to mental health difficulties, few effective service responses have been demonstrated.

As a mental health practitioner it is important to offer the best service to the client within the available resources. Small service changes may make great differences to the client. These can include the following.

- The opportunity for women to choose their keyworker or care manager (preference for male/female), and child care arrangements to enable women to use services they need (e.g. day hospital, outpatient clinics).
- Promotion of and liaison with women's agencies and groups which support local health provision (e.g. Women's Aid).

- Treatment responses targeted at issues that affect women.
- Staff training in women's issues.
- The involvement of women in service developments.

Many practitioners are women and as well as ensuring that appropriate resources are in place for female clients, there is a need to be aware of the challenges that prejudice the mental health of women using services.

WORKING BASE

Following the introduction of The Mental Health Act 1959 with its emphasis on reducing institutional care and developing community-based care, psychiatric services began to be set up in bases other than the traditional psychiatric hospitals. By the time the major report *Better Services for the Mentally Ill* (DHSS, 1975) was published, some psychiatric services were attached to district general hospitals or nurses were seconded out from the psychiatric institution. This report proposed the need to establish flexible and local services for the mentally ill with the specialist teams supporting the primary health care teams. Flexible responses to local needs have resulted in differences in the way these specialist mental health teams function and in the siting of their working bases. These differences should reflect locally assessed demand with the team being accessible to the users of the service. The mental health practitioners can therefore be based in a variety of settings which include the general hospital psychiatric unit, psychiatric day hospital or mental health centre.

With the advent of GP fundholding, attachment or secondment to GP surgeries and health centres is also taking place. The practitioner's working base may determine the nature and source of referrals, that is whether the majority of referrals come from primary sources such as the primary health care team or the specialist sources including the psychiatric wards and mental health care teams. Referrals from the ward will involve the practitioner in tertiary prevention, follow-up and aftercare. On the other hand, referrals from a health centre are more likely to involve the practitioner in secondary prevention, that is, decreasing the likelihood of admission (Simmons and Brooker, 1986).

Where the base is sited may also affect working relationships. For example, the practitioner may be directly attached to a multidisciplinary team in the same base, or a group of community psychiatric nurses may have a separate base from other disciplines. Liaison work, cross-referring, joint working and understanding of each other's role tends to be enhanced when working in a multidisciplinary setting. Wherever community mental health practitioners are based their flexible role and mobility means they are able to liaise between the hospital and the community and facilitate care continuity.

WORKING IN PARTNERSHIP – A COLLABORATIVE APPROACH TO CARE

In 1994 the Department of Health published a report of the mental health nursing review team. This was the first mental health nursing review since 1968 when it focused primarily on inpatient psychiatric nursing. The 1994 *Working in Partnership* Report (DoH, 1994d) reflects a fundamental shift in prevailing attitudes and philosophies of care with a drive towards community based services. To ensure the widest overview of mental health nursing the review team consulted and gained written and oral evidence from a number of sources. This included regional conferences, clinical practice areas, regional health authorities, district health authorities, family health service authorities, NHS trusts, mental health social services departments, community health councils, special health authorities, professional statutory bodies, individual practitioners, people who use the services and their carers, and other relevant agencies in the public, private and voluntary sectors.

It recommended that 'Mental health nursing should re-examine every aspect of its policy and practice in the light of the needs of people who use services' (DoH, 1994). To enable this to occur they identified 42 recommendations. It is important that all mental health nurses are aware of the recommendations as it is these recommendations that will be shaping the mental health services of the future of which they will be playing a part.

The recommendations are as follows.

1. We recommend that nurses improve their understanding and awareness of the racial and cultural needs of people who use services and ensure that these are fully reflected when developing care plans.
2. We recommend that mental health nurses take a lead role in ensuring that people in their care have access to appropriate information, including treatment options and rights.
3. We recommend that managers introduce a system of holding and acting upon information about people's wishes and needs in crisis.
4. We recommend the representation and participation of people who use services and their carers on service planning, education and research groups.
5. We recommend that the UKCC investigates and reports on the disproportionate numbers of disciplinary cases which involve male nurses and female patients.
6. We recommend that the essential focus for the work of mental health nurses lies in working with people with serious or enduring mental illness in secondary and tertiary care, regardless of setting.
7. We recommend that mental health nursing should retain its speciality at initial preparation level.

8. We recommend that care plans should be developed with individuals and based on their wishes and needs – not the convenience of the service.

9. We recommend that mental health nursing services should be arranged to ensure that nurses spend the majority of their time responding to the needs of people who use services.

10. We recommend that the title 'mental health nurse' be used both for nurses who work in the community and for those who work in hospital and day services.

11. We recommend that clinical supervision is established as an integral part of practice up to and including the level of advanced practitioner for mental health nurses.

12. We recommend that immediate action is taken to improve the standard of management and leadership in mental health nursing and mental health services.

13. We recommend that managers construct clear local strategies for mental health nursing, developing a framework for good practice.

14. We recommend that, in multidisciplinary/agency working, managers should establish protocols which explicitly define the relative responsibilities of the various professionals involved.

15. We recommend that commissioners and providers of mental health services include mental health nursing input when formulating, implementing and monitoring health care strategies.

16. We recommend the establishment of research programmes to examine the potential of liaison mental health nursing.

17. We recommend that mental health nursing skills are available to all members of the primary health care team and are directly accessible to the general public.

18. We recommend that action is taken to ensure that mental health nurses play a central role in services made available under the Care Programme Approach and in the provision of supervised discharge.

19. We recommend that the collective and individual needs of nurses presently working in large mental hospitals should be identified and met.

20. We recommend an urgent review of the therapeutic suitability of district general hospital mental health units.

21. We recommend that mental health services develop a system offering a choice of single-sex accommodation and gender of a keyworker.

22. We recommend a local review of the care currently being offered by mental health nurses to those suffering from HIV and other related diseases.

23. We recommend that a code of practice covering the issue of sexual harassment and abuse is developed for staff providing mental health services.

24. We recommend a local review of arrangements of the support and supervision of nurses working with elderly people with mental illness by commissioners and providers of mental health services.

25. We recommend a local review of the role and function of mental health nurses working in child and adolescent mental health services with a view to enabling them to work effectively alongside their colleagues, other disciplines and agencies.

26. We recommend that greater links are forged between mental health nurses working in substance misuse and services for mentally disordered offenders, and the criminal justice system.

27. We recommend that managers invest in the continuing developments of the research skills base among mental health nurses through a series of positive steps related to funded support.

28. We recommend that regional research and development committees define the action they are taking to respond to the recommendations of the task force on the strategy for research in nursing, midwifery and health visiting, with particular reference to mental health nursing.

29. We recommend that the Research and Development Division of the Department of Health identifies what mental health nursing research resources are at its disposal.

30. We recommend that a version of the Midwives Information Resource Service (MIDRIS) should be established for mental health nursing.

31. We recommend that the statutory bodies review the balance of time and emphasis given to each of the four branches within the Common Foundation Programme.

32. We recommend that people who use services and their carers should participate in teaching and curriculum development.

33. We recommend that teachers of mental health nursing should spend the equivalent of at least one day per week in practice to maintain the currency of their skills and knowledge.

34. We recommend that pre-registration education and training programmes ensure that students develop an awareness of the needs of those groups of people who are particularly vulnerable, such as homeless, unemployed and elderly people.

35. We recommend that all education and training programmes reflect the diversity of belief systems and cultural expectations that contribute to the life experience of people who use services.

36. We recommend a systematic national review of strategic planning to ensure that training commissions accurately reflect service needs.

37. We recommend that the period of rostered service within Project 2000 nursing programmes be discontinued.

38. We recommend that particular and appropriate education and training at post-registration level is made available for all mental health nurses.

39. We recommend that education providers should collaborate with service providers to develop further cost-effective shared learning packages which meet the needs of mental health nurses, other professionals and non-professional health care workers.

40. We recommend that action is taken to safeguard money available under Working Paper 10 arrangements.
41. We recommend that new training initiatives aimed at developing clinical supervision skills in senior clinical nurses are devised. We also recommend that newly qualified nurses and nursing students receive preparation in what to expect from clinical supervision.
42. We recommend that the United Kingdom Central Council for Nursing Midwifery and Health Visiting considers the accreditation of appropriate prior learning for entrants to pre-registration programmes.

The document itself offers a thorough investigation into mental health nursing at the present time.

For nurses to ensure that the recommendations take place and to give themselves full understanding of why the recommendations have come about it is necessary to read the full document. As the focus of mental health is now in the community it goes without saying that this is a particularly useful publication for all community practitioners.

Appendix

ORGANIZATIONS AND AGENCIES (NATIONAL)

Age Concern
1268, London Road
London SW16 4ER
0181 679 8000

Alcoholics Anonymous
61, Great Dover Street
London SE1
0171 403 0888

Alzheimers Disease Society
Gordon House
10, Greencoat Place
London SW1P 1PH
0171 306 0606 (helpline 0171 306 0833)

Carers National Association
20–25 Glasshouse Yard
London EC1A 4JS
0171 490 8898 (carers' line)

Cruse
Cruse House
126, Sheen Road
Richmond
TW9 1UR
0181 940 4818
0181 332 7227 (bereavement line)

Depressives Anonymous
36, Chestnut Avenue
Beverley
North Humberside
HW17 9QI
01482 860619

Eating Disorders Association
Sackville Place
44, Magdalen Place
Norwich NR3 1JU
01603 619090 (helpline 01603 621414)

Manic Depressive Fellowship
8–10, High Street
Kingston Upon Thames
Surrey
KT1 1EY
0181 974 6550

Mental Aftercare Association
25, Bedford Square
London WC1B 3HW
0171 436 6194

MIND
Granta House
15–19, Broadway
London E15 4BQ
0181 519 2122

Samaritans
10, The Grove
Slough SL1 1QP
01753 532 713 (helpline 0345 909090)

SANE
2nd Floor
199–205, Old Marylebone Road
London NW1 5QP
0171 724 6520

Tranquillizer, Anxiety and Stress Help Association
60, High Street
Brentford
Middlesex TW8 0AH
0181 569 9933

Zito Trust
P.O. Box 265
London WC2H 9JD
0171 240 0664

References

Appleby, M. (1992) Stress, in *A Textbook of Psychiatric and Mental Health Nursing*, (eds J. Brooking, S. Ritter and B. Thomas), Churchill Livingstone, Pearson Professional Ltd, Edinburgh.

Ackerman (1966) *Treating the Troubled Family*, Basic Books, New York.

Audit Commission for Local Authorities in England and Wales (1986) HMSO, London.

Bank-Mikkelson, N. (1979) The Danish Mental Retardation Service. Paper 1: The Quality of Care: Report of a Study Tour, London. National Society for Mentally Handicapped Children, London.

Barton, R. (1959) *Institutional Neurosis*, Wright, Bristol.

Beck, A.T. *et al.* (1961) Inventory for measuring depression, *Archives of General Psychiatry*, **4**, 561–71

Beck, A.T. and Emery, G. (1935) *Anxiety Disorders and Phobias: A Cognitive Perspective*, Basic Books, New York.

BMA (1996) *The British National Formulary*, British Medical Association and the Royal Pharmaceutical Society of Great Britain, London.

Bowlby, J. (1980) *Attachment and Loss Vol. III: Loss Sadness and Depression*, Hogarth Press, London.

Brooking, J. *et al.* (eds) (1992) *A Textbook of Psychiatric and Mental Health Nursing*, Churchill Livingstone, Pearson Professional Ltd, Edinburgh.

Brown, G. and Harris, T. (1978) *The Social Origins of Depression*, Tavistock Institute, London.

Burdick, M.B., Stuart, G.W. and Lewis, L.D. (1994) Measuring nursing outcomes in a psychiatric setting. *Issues in Mental Health Nursing* **15**(2), 137–48.

Butterworth, A. (1994) Preparing to take on clinical supervision. *Nursing Standard*, **8**, 32–4.

Caplan, G. (1961) *An Approach to Community Mental Health*, Tavistock Institute, London.

Carlisle, D. (1990) Are you accountable? *Nursing Times* 86–122.

Carson, J. *et al.* (1995) Stress and the CPN. *Community Psychiatric Nursing: a research perspective*, Vol. III (ed C. Brooker), Chapman & Hall, London.

Carpenter, D. (1993) Accountability in professional practice. In *Mental Health Nursing* (eds H. Wright and M. Giddey), Chapman & Hall, London.

Central Statistical Office (1984) *Social Trends*, HMSO, London.

Challis, D.J. (1990) Case management: problems and possibilities. In *Care Managers and Care Management* (ed T. Allen), Policy Studies Institute, London.

Cherniss, C. (1980) *Staff Burn out: Job Stress in the Human Services*, Sage, London.

Clare, A. (1976) *Psychiatry in Dissent*, Tavistock Publications, London.

Community Psychiatric Nurses Association (1980) *National Survey of Community Psychiatric Nursing Services*, CPNA Publications, Leeds.

Community Psychiatric Nurses Association (1985) *The 1985 CPNA National Survey Update*, CPNA Publications, Leeds.

Copp, L. (1986) The nurse as patient's advocate: pros and cons, *Nursing Mirror*, **11**, 138–40.

Crosby, P. (1989) *Quality Education System for the Individual. The Creative Factory*, McGraw-Hill, Maidenhead.

Crowcroft, A. (1967) *The Psychotic*, Penguin Books Limited, England.

Cumming, J. and Cumming, E. (1957) *Closed Ranks*, Harvard University Press, MA.

Dean, M. (1995) Alarm over supervised discharge orders. *The Lancet*, **345**, 4th March.

DHSS (1975) *Better Services for the Mentally Ill*, HMSO, London.

DHSS (1986) *Information and Guidance on AIDS (acquired immune deficiency syndrome)*, HMSO, London.

Dimond, B. (1990) *Legal Aspects of Nursing*, 2nd edn, Prentice Hall International (UK) Ltd, (Simon & Schuster International), Hemel Hempstead.

DoH (1990) *Care Programme Approach*, HMSO, London, HC(90), pp. 23–66.

DoH (1993a) *Code of Practice for the Mental Health Act*, 2nd edn, HMSO, London.

DoH (1993b) *A Vision for the Future*, NHS Management Executive, London.

DoH (1994a) *The Health of the Nation* 2nd edn, HMSO, London.

DoH (1994b) Introduction of supervision registers for mentally ill people from 1st April 1994, HSG(94)5, NHS Management Executive, London.

DoH (1994c) *Mental Illness Key Areas Handbook*, HMSO, London.

DoH (1994d) Working in partnership, *The Butterworth Report*, HMSO, London.

DoH (1995a) *The Health of the Nation. One Year on*, HMSO, London.

DoH (1995b) *The Patients' Charter*, 2nd edn, HMSO, London.

Donabedian, A. (1980) *The Definition of Quality and Approaches to its Assessment*, Vol. 1, Health Administration Press.

Egan, G. (1982) *The Skilled Helper*, 2nd edn, Brooks/Cole, Monterey.

Ellis, A. (1973) *Humanistic Psychotherapy, The Rational Emotive Approach*, Julian Press, New York.

English National Board (1989) *Health Promotion in Primary Health*, ENB, London.

Fottrell, E. (1983) *Case Histories in Psychiatry*, Churchill Livingstone, Pearson Professional Ltd, Edinburgh.

Freudenberger, H.J. (1974) Staff burn out. *Journal of Social Issues*, **30**(1), 159–66.

Gelder, M., Gath, D. and Mayou, R. (1994) *Concise Oxford Textbook of Psychiatry*, OUP, Oxford.

Gibbs, G. (1988) *Learning by Doing. A Guide to Teaching and Learning Methods*, Further Education Unit, Oxford Polytechnic, Oxford.

Gilbert, T. (1993) *Learning Disability Nursing: From Normalization to Materialism*, Routledge, London.

Goffman, E. (1961) *Asylums*, Penguin, Harmondsworth.

Goodman, J. (1984) Reflection and teacher education; a case study and theoretical analysis, *Interchange,* **15**(3), 9–26.

Green, S. (1991) Quality issues in mental health. *International Journal of Health Care Quality Assurance*, **4**(4), 15–16.

Griffiths, R. (1983) Why on earth do surgeons need quality assurance? Royal College of Surgeons, London, **70**, pp. 85–92.

Haley, J. (1976) *Problem Solving Therapy*, Jossey-Bass, San Francisco.

Harrison, K. (1995) Growing opposition to 'uncontroversial bill'. *Open Mind,* **74**.

Hawton, K. (1985) *Sex Therapy: A Practical Guide*, Oxford University Press, Oxford.

Health Advisory Service (1982) *The Rising Tide: developing services for mental illness in old age*, HAS, HMSO, London.

Heron, J. (1986) *Six Category Intervention Analysis*, 2nd edn, Human Resources Unit, University of Brighton.

Hershenson, D. and Power, P. (1987) *Mental Health Counselling*, Pergamon Press, Oxford.

Holmes, T. and Rahe, R. (1967) The social readjustment rating scale. *Journal of Psychosomatic Research*, **11**, 213–18.

Holsclaw, P. (1965) Nursing in high emotional risk areas. *Nursing Forum,* **4**(4), 36–45.

Hostick, T. (1995) A shared strategy (devising a quality assurance system for a community mental health team in East Yorkshire. *Nursing Standard,* **10**, 18th October, 21–2.

HSAC (1987) *Violence to Staff in the Health Care Services*, HMSO, London.

Hyde, P. (1985) Management accountability, *Nursing Mirror*, 3(16), 17–18 in *Journal of Advanced Nursing*, 1993, **18**, 1968–74.

Jarvis, P. (1992) *Adult and Continuing Education*, Routledge, London.

Johns, C. (1994) Nuances of reflection. *Journal of Clinical Nursing,* **3**, 271–5.

Jones, E.M. (1982) Who supports the nurse? in *Burn Out in the Nursing Profession* (ed E.A. McConnell), C V Mosby, St Louis.

Kempton, M. (1984) Family involvement; a planned reality orientation programme. *Nursing Mirror*, **159**, (18).

Kendall, H. (1988) The West Berkshire approach. *Nursing Times*, **84**(27), 33–4.

Kitson, A. (1985) *Standards of Care Project*, RCN, London.

Kitson, A. (1988) Raising the standards, *Nursing Times*, **84**(25), 38–42.

Kohner, N. (1994) *Clinical Supervision in Practice*, Kings Fund Centre, London.

Kucynski, J. (1980) Nursing and medical students sexual attitudes and knowledge. *Journal of Obstetric, Gynaecological and Neonatal Nursing*, Nov-Dec, 339–42.

Kumar, R. (1984) A study of emotional disorders in childbearing women. *British Journal of Psychiatry*, PTM Publishers Ltd, Surrey.

Lazarus, R. (1971) The concepts of stress and disease, in *Society, Stress and Disease Vol. 1, The Psycho Social Environment and Psychosomatic Disease*, (ed. L. Levis), Oxford University Press, London.

Lazarus, R. and Launier, R. (1978) Stress related transitions between person and environment in Maslac C. (1978) Job burn out, how people cope. *Public Welfare*, **36**, 56–8.

Lemert, E. (1967) *Human Deviance, Social Problems and Social Control*, Prentice Hall, New Jersey.

Maslac, C. (1979) Of the burn out syndrome and patient care, in *Stress and Survival – The Emotional Reality of Life Threatening Illness* (ed C.A. Garfield), C V Mosby, St Louis.

Maxwell, R.J. (1984) Quality assessment in health. *BMJ*, 12th May, 1470–2.

McCallion, H. (1991) Stress and nursing. University of Portsmouth. Dissertation.

Menzies, I.E.P. (1960) Nurse under stress. *International Nursing Review*, **7**(6), 9–16.

Mesibov, G. (1990) Normalization and its relevance today. *Journal of Autism and Developmental Disorders*, **20**(3), 379–91.

MIND (1992) *Stress on Women*, MIND, London.

MIND (1993) Policy on black and minority ethnic people and mental health, MIND, London.

Minuchin, S. (1974) *Families and Family Therapy*, Tavistock Institute, London.

Mullings, A.C. and Barstow, R.E. (1979) Care for the caretakers. *American Journal of Nursing*, August: 1425–7.

Myles, A. (1991) Psychology and health care, in *Nursing Practice and Health Care*, 2nd edn, (eds S. Hinchcliff, S. Norman and J. Schober, 1993), Edward Arnold, Hodder Headline, London.

Nelson, M. (1989) *Managing Health Professionals*, Chapman & Hall, London.

Nelson-Jones, R. (1988) *Practical Counselling and Helping Skills*, 2nd edn, Cassell, London.

NHS Training Directorate (1993) *Keeping the Record Straight*, HMSO, London.

NHS Training Division (1994) *Just for the Record*, HMSO, London.

NHS Training Directorate (1995) *Building on Strengths*, HMSO, London.

Nirje, B. (1969) The normalization principle and its human management implications, in *Changing Patterns in Residential Services for the Mentally Retarded* (eds R. Kugel and W. Wolfensberger), Washington US, The President's Committee on mental retardation, pp. 257–87.

O'Brien, J. (1987) *Framework for Accomplishment*, Responsive Systems Associates, Decatur, Georgia.

Onyett, S. (1994) *Case Management in Mental Health*, Chapman & Hall, London.

Ovreteit, J. (1993) *Co-ordinating Community Care*, Open University Press, Buckingham.

Parkes, C.M. (1972) *Bereavement: Studies of Grief in Adult Life*, Tavistock Institute, London.

Payne, M. (1986) *Social Care in the Community*, British Association of Social Workers, London.

Proctor, B. (1986) Supervision: a co-operative exercise in accountability, in *Enabling and Ensuring* (eds A. Marken and M. Payne), National Youth Bureau, Leicester.

Ramsey, R. (1979) Bereavement: a behavioural treatment for pathological grief, in *Trends in Behaviour Therapy* (eds P. Sivden *et al.*), Academic Press, New York.

Rhodes, B. (1983) Accountability in nursing. *Nursing Times*, **79**(36), 65–6.

Ritter, S. (1989) *Bethlem Royal and Maudsley Hospital Manual of Clinical Psychiatric Nursing Principles and Procedures*, Harper and Row, London.

Rogers, C. (1951) *Client Centred Therapy*, Houghton Mifflin, Boston.

Rogers, C. (1961) *On Becoming a Person*, Houghton Mifflin, Boston.

Rowden, L. (1993) Mind and body – the emotion and physical illness, in *Mental Health Nursing* (eds H. Wright and M. Giddey), Chapman and Hall, London.

Royal College of Nursing (1992) *Health of Half a Nation*, Royal College of Nursing, London.

Royal College of Psychiatrists (1989) *HIV Disease and Psychiatric Practice*, RCP, London.

Sale, D. (1991) *Essentials of Nursing Management: Quality Assurance*, MacMillan, Basingstoke.

Scheff, R. (1966) *Being Mentally Ill*, Weidenfeld & Nicolson, London.

Schmadl, J.C. (1979) Quality assurance: examination of the concept. *Nursing Outlook*, 27(7), 462–5.

Seligman, M. (1975) *Helplessness: On Depression, Development and Death*, Freeman, San Francisco.

Selye, H. (1956) *The Stress of Life*, McGraw Hill, New York.

Simmons, S. (1984) Family burden. What does it mean to the carers? University of Surrey. Dissertation.

Simmons, S. and Brooker, C. (1986) *Community Psychiatric Nursing*, Heinemann Nursing, Oxford.

Simmons, S. and Morrisey, J. (1995) Community mental health nursing, in *Current Issues in Community Nursing* (ed. J. Littlewood), Churchill Livingstone, Pearson Professional Ltd, London.

Spaniel, L. and Capputo, J. (1978) *Professional Burnout: a personal survival kit*, Human Service Association, Lexington, Mass.

Street (1991) From image to action. *Reflection in Nursing Practice*. Deaking University Press, Geelong, Australia.

Stuart, G. and Sundeen, S. (1995) *Principles and Practice of Psychiatric Nursing*, 5th edn, C V Mosby, St Louis.

Sugden, J. *et al*, (1986) *A Handbook for Psychiatric Nurses*, Harper and Row, London.

Tingle, J. (1990) Responsible and liable. *Nursing Times*, 86(25), 42–3.

Tschudin, V. (1986) *Ethics in Nursing*, Heinemann, London.

UKCC (1984a) *Code of Professional Conduct for the Nurse, Midwife and Health Visitor*, UKCC, London.

UKCC (1984b) *Scope for Professional Practice*, UKCC, London.

UKCC (1986) *Project 2000: a new preparation for practice*, UKCC, London.

UKCC (1989) *Exercising Accountability*, UKCC, London.

UKCC (1993) *Standards for Records and Record Keeping*, UKCC, London.

US Department of Health and Human Services (1988) Update: universal precautions for prevention of transmission of human immunodeficiency virus, *Morbidity and Mortality Weekly Report*, 37(24), 377–82.

Verbrugge, L.M. (1985) Gender and health. *Journal of Health and Social Behaviour*, 26, 156–82, in *Sociology of Health and Health Care* (eds S. Taylor and D. Field, 1993), Blackwell Scientific Publications, London.

Walker, D. (1985) Writing and reflection, in *Reflection: Turning Experience into Learning* (eds D. Bond, D. Keogh and D. Walker), Kogan Page, London.

Ward, M. (1985) *The Nursing Process in Psychiatry*, Churchill Livingstone, Pearson Professional Ltd, Edinburgh.

White, N. and Watt, K. (1981) *The Abnormal Personality*, John Wiley, Chichester.

Whittington R. and Wykes, T. (1994) The prediction of violence in a health care setting, in *Violence and Health Care* (ed. T. Wykes), Chapman & Hall, London.

Wolfensberger, W. (1972) *The Principle of Normalisation in Human Services,* National Institute of Mental Retardation, Toronto.

World Health Organization (1981) *Global Strategy for Health for All by the Year 2000,* WHO, Geneva.

World Health Organization (1985) WHO Euro Reports – the principles of quality assurance, WHO Regional Office for Europe, Copenhagen.

Further reading

Argyle, M. and Trower, P. (1979) *Person to Person: Ways of Communicating*, Harper and Row, London.

Babcock, D. and Miller, M. (1994) *Client Education: Theory and Practice*, C V Mosby, London.

Bloch, D. (1980) Interrelated issues in evaluation and evaluation research: a researcher's perspective, *Nursing Researcher,* 29(2), 69–73.

Bond, S. and Thomas, L. (1991) Issues in measuring outcomes of nursing. *Journal of Advanced Nursing,* 16, 1492–523.

Brown, T., Scott, A. and Pullen, I. (1990) *Handbook of Emergency Psychiatry*, Churchill Livingstone, Pearson Professional Ltd, London.

Cherniss, D. (1990) *Staff Burn Out: Job Stress in the Human Services*, Sage, London.

Cole, F. and Slocumb, E. (1993) Nurses' attitudes towards patients with Aids. *Journal of Advanced Nursing*, 18, 1112–17.

Department of Health (1989) *Caring for People*, HMSO, London.

DHSS (1981) The primary health care team, *The Harding Report*, HMSO, London.

Dingwall, R. *et al.,* (1988) *An Introduction to the Social History of Nursing*, Routledge, London.

DoH (1990) *NHS and Community Care Act (1990)*, HMSO, London.

Duggirala, C. *et al.* (1995) Schizophrenia and Downs syndrome. *Irish Journal of Advanced Nursing,* 17, 561–8.

Johns, C. (1990) Autonomy for primary nurses: the need to both facilitate and limit autonomy in practice. *Journal of Advanced Nursing*, 15, 886–94.

Johns, L. (1990) Setting standards: steps to self medication. *Nursing Times,* 86(16), 46–9.

Kitson, A. (1987) A comparative analysis of day-caring and professional (nursing) caring relationships. *International Journal of Nursing Studies*, 24(2), 155–65.

Lambert, C. (1994) Depression (Part 2) Nursing management. *Nursing Standard*, 8(48).

NHS Training Division (1995) *Developing the Care Programme Approach*, HMSO, London.

NHSEF (1994) *Local Systems of Support*, HMSO, London.

Royal Commission on the National Health Service (1979) *The Merrison Report*, HMSO, London.

Ryan, A. (1993) Therapeutic risks in mental health nursing. *Nursing Standard*, 7(24).

Sale, D. (1988) Down Dorset Way. *Nursing Times*, **84**(28), 31–3.

Stacey, M. (1988) *A Sociology of Health and Healing*, Routledge, London.

Sumpter, J., Ryan, C. and Holmes-Smith, S. (1993) Mind, body and soul. *Nursing Times*, **89**(23).

Taylor, S. and Field, D. (eds) (1993) *Sociology of Health and Health Care*, Blackwell Scientific Publications, Oxford.

The North East Thames and The South East Thames Health Authority (1994) *The Report of the Inquiry into the Care and Treatment of Christopher Clunis*, HMSO, London.

Thompson, I. *et al.* (1988) *Nursing Ethics*, Churchill Livingstone, Pearson Professional Ltd, Edinburgh.

Townsend, P., Davison, N. and Whitehead, M. (1988) *Inequalities in Health: The Black Report/The Health Divide*, Penguin Books, Harmondsworth.

Van Maanenm, H.M. (1985) Evaluation of nursing care, in *Measuring the Quality of Care* (eds L.D. Willis and M. Linwood, 1984), Churchill Livingstone, Pearson Professional Ltd, Edinburgh.

Waters, H. (1987) All for one and one for all. *Nursing Times*, 6th May, Vol. 83.

Wright, D. (1984) An introduction to the evaluation of nursing care. *Journal of Advanced Nursing*, **9**, 457–67.

Wright, H. and Giddey, M. (eds) (1993) *Mental Health Nursing*, Chapman & Hall, London.

Wykes, T. (1993) *Violence and Health Care Professionals*, Chapman & Hall, London.

Yalom, I. (1985) *Principles and Practice of Group Psychotherapy*, Basic Books, New York.